RAW ADDICTION

Easy, Delicious & Addictive Recipes to Reverse Ageing and Disease

By Katrina Ellis N.D.
Naturopath, Iridologist, Herbalist, Lecturer

Copyright © Katrina Ellis 2012

This book is copyright. Except for private study, research, criticism or reviews, as permitted under the Copyright Act, no part of this book may be reproduced, stored in a retrieval system or transmitted in any form or by any means without prior written permission. **Enquiries should be made to Ellis-Crawford Media, Shop 2,/60 Musgrave Street, Kirra, Qld 4225, Australia.**
www.katrinaellis.com.au/

This book or any information contained within is not intended to treat, diagnose or cure and is not to take the place of medical advice or treatment. This book is a work of non-fiction. The author asserts her moral rights.

Legal Deposit Lodgment: (In accordance with the Copyright Act 1968)
National Library of Australia
State Library of Queensland

Cataloguing-in-Publication Data available on request
National Library of Australia
Author: Katrina Ellis
Title: Raw Addiction/ 1st Edition
ISBN: 978-0-9874669-1-4

© Cover Design – Major Print Burleigh Heads 2012
© Photography – Brian Usher, Ocean Road Magazine

Published with the assistance of
Publicious Pty Ltd
www.publicious.com.au

CONTENTS ...

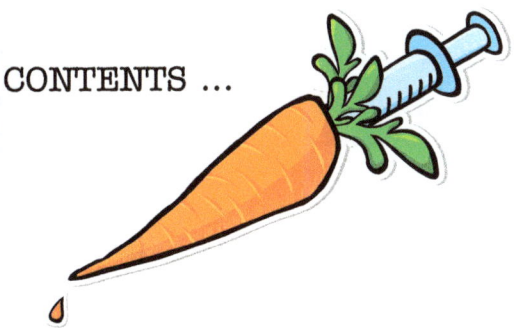

Introduction   6
My Journey Back Towards Living Foods
Living Foods VS Raw Foods
The Perfect Diet for You
The Healing Potential of Raw Foods
Fresh Organics = Happy Planet
My Kitchen Tools
The Power of Sprouting
Shopping Checklist
How to Use this Book

Power Drinks for Radiant Health   32
Nutty Milks
Super Fruit Smoothies
Green Smoothie Madness
'Shake It Up' Power Drinks
Juices

56   **Breakfast Ideas**
Super Yummy Cereals
Breakfast Whips and Yoghurts
Breakfast Scrambles

70   **Breads, Crackers and Chips**
Healthy Breads
Crackers and Chips
Raw Pizza Bases

82   **Scrumptious Sauces and Spreads**
Fantastic Fillings
Scrumptious Sauces and Spreads
Delicious Dips
Mock Cheese
Salad Dressings

114   **Nourishing Soups**

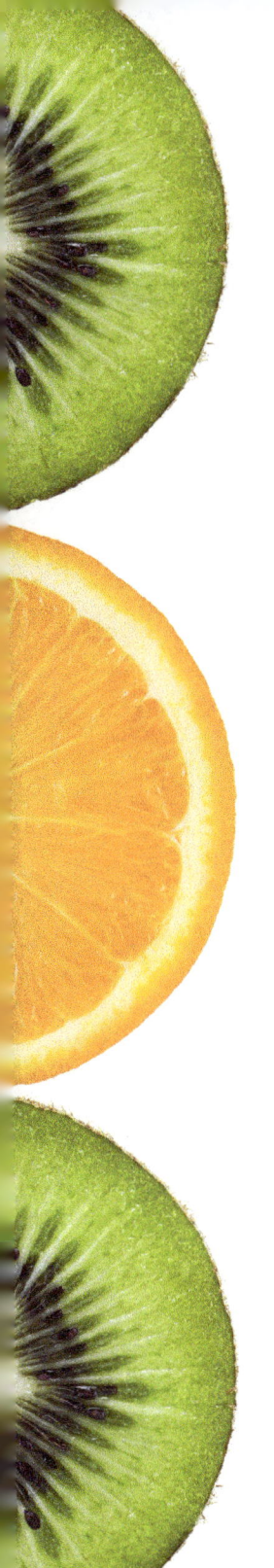

Salads with Punch — 126

Mains to Die For — 144
Pasta with Passion
Guilt Free Burgers
Burrito Cups
Mock Sushi
Curry in a Hurry
More Mains to Die For

Not so Naughty Sweet Treats — 166
Creamy Treats and Ice-Dreams
Cakes and Pies
Super Slices and Chocolate Indulgence

Back of the Book — 182
My Shopping List

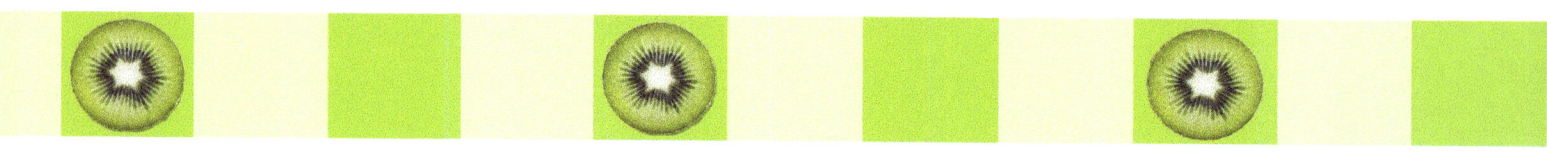

Introduction ..

Addiction to saturated fats, sugar, processed, and other nasty foods is on the rise and with it is the rise of 'modern diseases' like arthritis, diabetes, obesity and cancer. People always ask me 'why is cancer so common today?' The answer to this question isn't 'rocket science'. Our food, which is meant to be the substance that fuels and heals our body is tainted from the moment the seed is put into the ground. The soil where the seed is grown contains no anti-cancer or healing minerals. By the time the vegetable, fruit or grain begins to grow it is sprayed with a toxic concoction of fertilizers and herbicides to enhance its growth. It is then picked, stored, processed and altered with dangerous additives, preservatives and colourings to make it more appealing to the public eye and our now desensitized taste buds. By the time the original food reaches you on your plate it is no longer a 'living food' anymore, but rather a 'toxic science experiment' designed to wreak havoc and cause destruction within your body.

One of my greatest aims in creating 'Raw Addiction' was to draw people back towards the simplicity of 'living foods' and in doing so help to reverse modern day illness and disease. The only way to truly do this is to get people addicted to the tantalizing taste and variety of 'raw and living foods'. It took me so long to write 'Raw Addiction' as I had to make sure that all one hundred and fifty recipes were packed full of flavour, nutrition and healing impact. You don't have to be a 'master chef' to make these healing creations – all you need is a good food processor and ten minutes of your time. When you taste the recipes in 'Raw Addiction' it will be hard to believe that you are actually eating raw.

Within nature's foods are the complex answers to reversing disease. I have beaten malignant cancer and overcome infertility with the help of nature's foods. Over the past twenty years of practicing natural medicine I have personally witnessed people with serious health conditions like asthma, lupus, diabetes, autism, ADD and cancer reverse their mysterious ailments simply by returning back towards a traditional, living foods diet. To many people this sounds too easy and without doubt, most people are looking for a 'quick fix' to their ailment in the form of a 'medicine or drug'. But when you consider the fact that a poor diet was most likely the cause of your health condition, doesn't it make sense that a good diet would be the answer to reverse your ailment. This book is a 'living food resource' for anyone who wishes to live a healthier and happier life. My children love the recipes in 'Raw Addiction' especially the mock choc nutty milks, the sun burgers and the super food truffles. Little do they know their chocolate truffles are laced with green super foods and their nutty milks are actually mineral rich nuts, seeds and herbs – all secret remedies to enhance their learning, behavior, growth and happiness.

Many women in today's world want to lose weight, slow down ageing and improve their physical beauty. I am a girl who loves to take care of her physical appearance so I completely understand a woman's desire to look more beautiful on the outside. This book gives you the tools to rejuvenate your cells on the inside, so you glow with radiance and beauty on the outside. I have balanced all of my living food recipes in healing value to ensure you will receive the perfect nutrients to feel younger, happier and healthier within a few weeks. Every creation is designed to be not only delicious, but to enhance and transform health and well-being, on both an emotional and physical level.

'Raw Addiction' can benefit every facet of your life, without the need for pills, potions or quick fixes. The answer to authentic health, beauty, vitality and inner peace lies in the magic of earth's living foods and within these pages I am offering you the secrets that I use daily to stay youthful, vibrant and fit both mentally and physically. By getting addicted to the 'power of raw foods' you will not only be transforming your health and the people you love, but also saving the future of our 'living, green planet' in the process.

my journey back towards living foods ...

Since I was a little girl I have always been fascinated by the healing power of food. My life has been surrounded by good food, healthy exercise and outdoor activities. My father was a very talented sportsman – he skillfully played and coached football, boxing, athletics, swimming and even gymnastics - you name it and my father could do it. For many years he was a top fitness instructor in the Australian army so his health and physique was always at peak levels. My mother was very new age in many ways. She began reading Adelle Davis and Ruth Cilento when I was a little girl and visited top nutritionists to find out the best food for herself, her husband and her family. I remember going to school and all of my friends were eating white bread sandwiches, while I would open my lunchbox to wholemeal salad sandwiches, organic fruit and spelt muffins. So being surrounded by healthy foods and an active outdoor lifestyle definitely had a powerful impact in ensuring that I would fulfill the direction and passion of my life.

At a young age I became a champion sprinter and I excelled in any sport I tried. After travelling Australia and seeing the beauty of my country, my heart had a strong urge to study natural medicine, nutrition and herbalism. Even though my father always provided a secure environment for me to live, he taught me that it was important to work as it would give me the confidence and experience to achieve whatever my heart desired. Fortunately I found a great job working for one of Australia's best raw food and vegan cooks. David and his wife were instrumental in setting up some of the best raw food restaurants in Australia including the 'Garden of Eden' on the Gold Coast. At the age of nineteen I was taught about the diversity of living foods. When I would open the shop, Max the 'salad genius' would turn his music up as loud as possible and begin pumping out not only tunes, but some of the most amazing raw salad creations I have ever seen. He taught me how to make living foods full of flavour! He could make the healthiest living food into a pure taste sensation. In an instant he would whip up an incredible salad from black sesame seeds, red capsicum, watercress and sprouts topped with soy and honey marinated tofu chunks dripping in lemon and ginger sauce. Simply delicious, yet totally nutritious in every way. Pattie and Sharon, the 'hot food magicians' would brew up a storm of curried dhal with wild rice, polenta balls with tomato salsa, vegan spinach pies and nutmeg rolls – all vegan, dairy free and completely delicious. I had no idea 'living foods' could taste so good. This amazing team of 'living food enthusiasts' taught me how to combine herbs and spices to create flavour and balance in foods that were normally considered bland. I would work in the front of the shop experimenting with juices, smoothies, healthy wraps, vegan burgers and so much more, but secretly I loved to sneak into the back of the shop to learn how to create raw food sensations. This real-life experience combined with studying natural medicine ignited an even greater passion within me to learn about the healing power of living foods.

After finishing my studies, I was fortunate to secure an amazing job in Thailand working for the ex-deputy prime minister in his five star health resort, Chiva-Som. Here I was employed as head naturopath, nutritionist and yoga instructor, as well as 'health food consultant' to the Thai chefs. I suddenly found myself in a strange exotic land working as the only westerner amongst hundreds of Thai employees. The Thai chefs had never been taught about the nutritional value of foods and how certain foods could enhance detoxification, rejuvenation and healing. This is no disrespect to the Thai people, as their diet is quite incredible with its rich assortment of fresh seafood, herbs, spices, fruits, seeds and vegetables. But when you are expected to design detoxification and weight loss programs for celebrities and hydrogenated coconut milk, raw sugar, sodium rich fish sauce and corn flakes are on the menu, then your ability to achieve these goals are definitely hindered. So, at the age of twenty-two, I was designated the job of creating health food menus for in-house dining and detoxification, and weight loss and rejuvenation programs to meet the health goals of guests from all over the world. Fortunately, I had knowledge from my studies and experience from working with some of the best raw food guru's in the world. I began teaching the Thai chefs about healthy traditional foods and how to swap ingredients like white sugar for apple juice concentrate and fish sauce for tamari or celtic salt. I designed a successful '3 day detoxification cleanse' using fresh fruits, juices and vegetable broths. The daily breakfast items changed from packaged cereals and fried eggs to home-made muesli, stewed apples with prunes, fresh juices and fruits, home-made puddings, miso soup and more. Working together we designed a range of organic food products sold throughout Thailand and a recipe book that was internationally acclaimed. My love for living foods and how these could integrate with traditional Thai and Asian foods become stronger every day.

After living in this beautiful paradise for many years, my body began to break down. Overwork, a bad relationship, a radical change in diet, and exposure to a toxic agent finally broke down my defenses. At the age of 27 I had developed a rare and aggressive form of malignant cancer. In a few months the tumour had grown to the size of a small baby, and after several mis-diagnoses I eventually had the tumour removed, but not before it had spread. Young, scared and afraid of dying, I caved in to having large amounts of chemotherapy pumped into my veins. Luckily my journey had not diminished my belief in healing foods, so during this challenging fight for my life, I incorporated living foods back into my diet. Even if I felt sick and tired, I juiced organics, made power shakes, vegetable miso soups and ate any food that I knew had a potent cancer-fighting potential. After almost 90 hours of chemotherapy, my life force was drained and my body had reached its limit. I knew it, but the doctors kept insisting that I press on, even though I had dangerously low white blood cells. I drew on every ounce of strength to grab the courage to STOP treatment and find my body's healing potential once again.

I knew that the answer to my survival lay in my knowledge and experience with nature's foods and plants. Courageously I said 'no more' and, with the support of my parents and faithful juicer/blender, I began indulging in the magic of 'living foods' to save my life. Day by day I became stronger and healthier and my skin and eyes began to glow with vitality. I could smell the toxic chemicals seeping from my pores as the clean, living foods flooded my body with healing substances. Of course I used the power of my mind to help this healing process, I knew in my heart I could win and I never doubted this, but at the INTEGRAL heart of all of this was the secret cancer-fighting elements found in nature's foods. As soon as I felt rejuvenated I made the choice to visit my specialist – not because I wanted reassurance, but because I wanted him to know how I had beaten this, perhaps hoping within my mind that he could pass this knowledge onto others. He looked at my results and in a pleasant detached manner said "There doesn't seem to be any cancer. But just to let you know, this type of cancer definitely returns and you could still be dead within a year. And, it is not likely that you will ever have children'. Most people would have been shocked by these comments, but I am not one of those. It simply made me more determined to prove that he was wrong.

Instead of choosing to live a life with the 'fear of my cancer returning' I chose a completely different path, enjoying each moment by indulging in my passions of surfing, writing and anything connected to nature, including natural medicine and healthy, living foods. I released the international best seller 'Shattering the Cancer Myth' written to empower individuals in their fight against cancer. With the power of natural medicine and the love of my husband we created two tiny natural miracles in the form of a beautiful boy and girl. I continued to work with clients from all over the world suffering from all types of health imbalances. After working with thousands of patients I came to the conclusion that 'a traditional, living diet' is the most important key to prevent and rectify most diseases.

My journey with nature's foods began when I was a child and it is still continuing to this day. I have been surrounded by the power of natural medicine and living foods for over thirty years. I have beaten a malignant form of cancer and overcome the possibility of not having children. My greatest ally in my fight to reclaim wellness was not only the power of my mind, but nature's healing foods. This book is a culmination of years of experience and wisdom, not only of my own, but also of the countless brave souls and healers that have touched my life. Within this book are the 'living food tools' to guide you back towards vitality, longevity and ideal health. I originally developed this book to help individuals overcome cancer, but in its creation it has become a living resource to help anyone find their perfect weight, vitality and radiant beauty once again. I have tested and created every recipe within this book to ensure they are delicious, easy to make and balanced in nutritional value and healing potential. The secret to reversing disease and reclaiming your authentic weight, energy and beauty is found within these pages and the magic of nature's living foods.

living foods VS raw foods ...

I do not believe that LIVING foods are the same as RAW foods, even though the words are used interchangeably. Any food from the earth which is fresh and unheated is a living food. Even though I have a dehydrator and I know how to use this to create 'dehydrated foods', I don't use this very often, as I try not to heat any 'living food' above a certain temperature to ensure the enzymes and living nutrients are unharmed. Otherwise, I would rather eat the food completely raw. Living foods contain lots of enzymes. Enzymes are the spark plugs or catalysts for hundreds of biochemical reactions within the human body including energy, immunity, thinking, digestion and even cell repair. They are the 'turning keys' to reversing complex diseases.

Some foods may be classed 'raw', but they do not contain any enzyme potential. For example, a 'raw cracker' can be dehydrated so long that it has undergone fermentation and contains no water content. This makes it difficult to digest, draws valuable water from body organs to balance out the dryness and places extra stress on the digestive system. Another example of this is a legume or nut. When it is soaked and sprouted it is much higher in nutrient potential than an un-soaked nut or legume. The 'raw food' which was un-soaked, has now become a 'living food', which has been soaked, higher in enzyme potential. Therefore, living foods are different to raw foods.

Living foods contain the ingredients to reignite a cell's repair mechanism and in the process prevent and reverse many confusing and mysterious diseases. Without enzymes found in living foods, human life would cease to exist. To get the full benefit of the 'healing life force' found within foods, it is beneficial to eat a combination of both raw and living foods.

the perfect diet for you ...

The easiest and cheapest way to reclaim wellness is to begin adding living foods with the greatest healing potential into your diet. As powerful as nutritional supplements are, they cannot identically replicate the perfection found within nature's foods. It is within a plant that countless healing nutrients are found, each with their own potential to heal and to synergistically improve the absorption of other nutrients found within the plant. When choosing produce it is important to source these from nutrient rich organic soils. A plant flourishes with the help of water, soil and sunlight – absorbing its energy to convert this into a vast powerhouse of healing nutrients. If the soil, water or sunlight is filled with pesticides or pollution, then the plant will absorb these toxic poisons and when you eat the fruit, vegetable, nut or seed you are also partaking in the toxic warehouse that was used on the plant. Many people believe 'organic' is simply too expensive to buy. In these cases, I would suggest buying anything open leaf in an organic form, like lettuces, spinach, broccoli, cauliflower, blueberries and so on. If you are still unable to buy organic, why not try growing your own pesticide-free herbs and vegetables or seek out produce from local farmers or co-op's. Many practitioners believe that a purely 'raw foods' diet is the only answer to cure disease. I do believe raw foods can reverse illness, but I also believe that a purely raw foods diet does not suit every situation. If an individual is malnourished or underweight, a completely raw foods diet would cause them to lose too much weight. Cooked foods are easier to digest when a person is in a weakened state. In these cases, around 75% raw foods would be ideal, in combination with hot soups, steamed vegetables, local fish (from small fishing boats) and eggs to maintain life force, muscle strength and vitality. It is also a great way to obtain protein and omega 3 fatty acids to enhance immunity and decrease inflammation.

Likewise some constitutions do not thrive on a purely vegan diet. Many vegans can be prone to developing iron, protein and Vitamin B12 deficiencies. The best way to overcome this is by eating more fermented foods like organic natto, tempeh and tofu or using hemp seed protein, nutritional yeast, algae and similar substances. Even though these sources claim to have Vitamin B12, some research indicates that levels are negligible and poorly absorbed. Vitamin B12 is important as it helps with red blood cell production and a deficiency can cause dizziness, fatigue, constipation, shortness of breath, nervous system disorders and even cancer.

To find the ideal balance of foods that perfectly suits your genetic make-up, I think it important to be grounded and non-fanatical in your approach. There are hundreds of weight loss diets preying on the insecurities of women to become thinner and more beautiful like unrealistic magazine models. The problem with most of these high protein or liquid diets, is that once you return to eating normally you pack the weight on worse than before. These diets never consider long-term wellness or disease prevention. For example, if I decided to eat a purely protein diet, eventually my kidneys would become overworked, my acidity levels would rise and protein will leech into my bloodstream causing fatigue, fluid retention and toxicity. In the short term I will definitely lose weight quickly, but what about the long-term impact on my health? I believe the most successful eating plan to achieve your beauty or weight loss goals is to return back towards a traditional, living foods diet. While writing this book I dined only on the recipes within 'Raw Addiction'. Within one month I returned to my perfect pre-baby weight even trimming down my tummy fat, my skin glowed with youth, my hair became luscious and grew quickly and my energy was beyond belief. I literally stripped years off my biological age. And to top this off, I slept beautifully, woke with energy and found myself alert, creative and in a perfect state to manifest my heart's desires. The answer to true health, beauty and vitality lies in the magic of earth's living foods and I am now offering you the secrets that I use daily to stay youthful, vibrant and fit both mentally and physically.

healing potential of raw foods ...

Have you ever seen an overweight lion or cheetah living in the jungle? What about an chubby ladybug or an obese orangutan? A sight like this would definitely be quite peculiar to see. This is because animals which live in our 'natural world' only feed on living, raw foods found within nature. And by doing so they stay at a perfect weight and maintain constant energy levels to be able to prey, feed and mate successfully. We could certainly learn some great lessons from our animal counterparts. Instead we choose to spray, store, enhance, cook and process every type of natural food, leaving us with toxic, devitalized food that lacks any nutritional value. Eating dead foods are a great way to advance the ageing process, drain energy levels and clog up our arteries, colon and detoxification organs. Dead foods should be put on trial for causing the death of millions of people from cancer, heart disease and diabetes. I believe most diseases can be prevented and I also believe that the majority of these are linked to dietary causes.

A diet rich in fresh fruits and vegetables, nuts, seeds and legumes is not only full of healing nutrients, it is also naturally alkaline in nature. When the body is highly acidic, diseases like arthritis, asthma, eczema, psoriasis, chronic fatigue and even cancer begin to thrive. By switching to a primarily vegetarian, raw foods diet the body slowly becomes more alkaline. Raw foods are easy to digest and deliver large amounts of healing value with very minimal effort. Studies have shown that living foods contain enough healing potential to overcome many illnesses. Research and real life stories have proven that a person can prevent healthy cells from turning into cancerous cells simply by consuming a predominantly raw foods diet. Fresh organic living foods contain high amounts of WATER and OXYGEN. Water is the 'elixir of all life'. Our blood is eighty per cent water. Water obtained from fresh fruits and vegetables flushes toxins from the body and rehydrates cells to ensure superb energy and lymphatic, kidney, digestive and liver function. Without water, nutrition is unable to be delivered to body organs to ensure their optimal function and repair mechanisms. Oxygen is imperative to all existence and it is now becoming a restricted commodity with more urban growth and a higher amount of logging and pollution, resulting in less oxygen from fewer trees. Oxygen is found in good amounts in uncooked foods. Remember, cancer cells, bacteria, yeast and parasites find it impossible to live in oxygenated environments, so by flooding the body with oxygenated raw foods, you are also flooding the body with oxygen to wipe out nasty cells.

Raw foods are abundant in natural FIBRE. Fibre acts like a broom sweeping through the colon removing heavy metals, toxins, bad hormones and cholesterol. This not only protects against heart disease, it also offers valuable protection against colon, breast and liver cancer. Removing toxins and unwanted hormones via the bowels, takes the strain off the liver, allowing it to do more important jobs of filtration, energy production and cholesterol maintenance. If the liver receives less toxins from the bowels, it is able to filter beautiful clean blood to every tissue, cell and body organ. ENZYMES are the spark plugs of human life that rejuvenate cells and repair damage. The more enzymes you have, the quicker you can re-create younger, healthier and stronger cells. Enzymes are able to break down fibrin coatings surrounding tumours, allowing your own white blood cell immune warriors better access to destroying tumours. Enzymes are found abundantly within living, raw foods. ANTIOXIDANTS prevent damage to cells caused from free radicals. Free radicals are dangerous substances that have been implicated in countless diseases including cancer, heart disease and advanced ageing. Nature's living foods contain huge amounts of antioxidants to reverse and repair cell damage that can lead to disease and advanced ageing. Some fresh fruits contain up to eighteen different antioxidants.

The foods in this book are based on my own personal experience in beating terminal cancer, as well as many years of working as an international naturopath, iridologist and herbalist. Living organic foods high in healing value was my most IMPORTANT tool in beating cancer and overcoming infertility. I always tell my clients that as powerful as supplements are they will not work successfully without the right foods. Whole living foods supply the body with live enzymes, antioxidants and phytonutrients that cannot be identically replicated in supplement form. A simple addition of raw, living foods into your diet will allow you to experience more vitality, youthfulness and a better bank balance from fewer trips to the doctor. On top of this, you will need less sleep, wake with more energy and maintain a perfect body weight. If you still think that raw foods could not have such a powerful impact on your health, then why not try it out for yourself. I think you will be surprised at how quickly your body adapts to a diet that resonates with the ancient memory of its soul.

fresh organics = happy planet ...

Organic foods are thought to be at least ten times greater in nutritional value than non-organic produce. A two year study on strawberries showed that organic strawberries were not only more delicious but far greater in nutritional content than their sprayed counterparts. This may shock you, but some vegetables and fruits are grown with the use of over fifty different pesticides and herbicides, with strawberries, blueberries and broccoli close to the top of the list. A report produced by the Organic Center and Professors from the University of Florida Department of Horticulture and Washington State University provided evidence that organic foods contain on average 25 percent higher concentration of 11 important nutrients, compared to their sprayed counterparts. True organics are grown in mineral-rich soils which ensures that huge amounts of nutrition are passed through to the plant and then on to YOU.

Pesticides and herbicides kill minerals within the soils by destroying beneficial organisms needed for healthy soil. Dead, infertile soil equates to dead, devitalized produce. Pesticide exposure has been linked to lymphoma, leukemia, autism, cancer, autoimmune conditions and neurological and developmental problems in children. In my practice I work closely with cancer patients. Many of my clients have grown up in areas exposed to high amounts of dangerous pesticides and herbicides and without doubt, there are belts of cancer cases in these farming areas. By supporting organics, you are supporting the earth and reducing the 'dangerous chemical mess' left in the soils that will eventually harm our animals, children and our chance of a beautiful clean and disease free future. By supporting organics, you will help to ensure that organic farmers continue to expand and provide clean produce for every individual at a more competitive price.

my kitchen tools ...

There are certain tools that are essential in a 'living kitchen' to not only make delicious raw dishes, but to make the food quickly and simply. The most important ingredient is a good blender or food processor. You can buy these separately, but I believe it is worth the investment to purchase a good food processor/blender in one. My recommendations are based on experience, not endorsement. There are some great blenders out there like the vitamix, powermill, blendtec or thermomix. I use a vitamix in my kitchen because it is very reliable and blends beautifully while leaving the enzymes unharmed. If your budget is an issue, there are some cheaper options available and I am constantly looking out for new blenders that are efficient and affordable.

The next tool can be important if you wish to heat foods or dehydrate snacks. I use the Excalibur dehydrator – it is brilliant as it has a number of different layers for dehydrating. Make sure you buy one that has a timer on it to ensure that you won't have to keep an eye on the food all of the time. I think it is important to purchase some teflex sheets with this to make pizza bases, cookies and anything you don't want to stick to the mesh trays. I don't use my dehydrator all the time, but there are times when I feel like making live breads, crackers, pizza bases and chips and then I will use for days in a row. You can always start with a blender/food processor and when you are completely addicted to the brilliance of raw foods, invest in a dehydrator.

The next tool which isn't essential, but I love to use is a spiralizer. It turns vegetables into brilliant spaghetti or noodle strands for raw pasta and noodle dishes. My kids love using this as it makes raw food fun and interesting. The spiralizer is now being superseded by the spirooli – so my spiralizer has taken a back seat to the ease, function and versatility of my new spirooli. It turns vegetables into lots of different noodle strands, garnishings and shapes – I simply love it. My kids love making noodles on the spirooli and it makes them love their raw carrots and other vegie's even more.

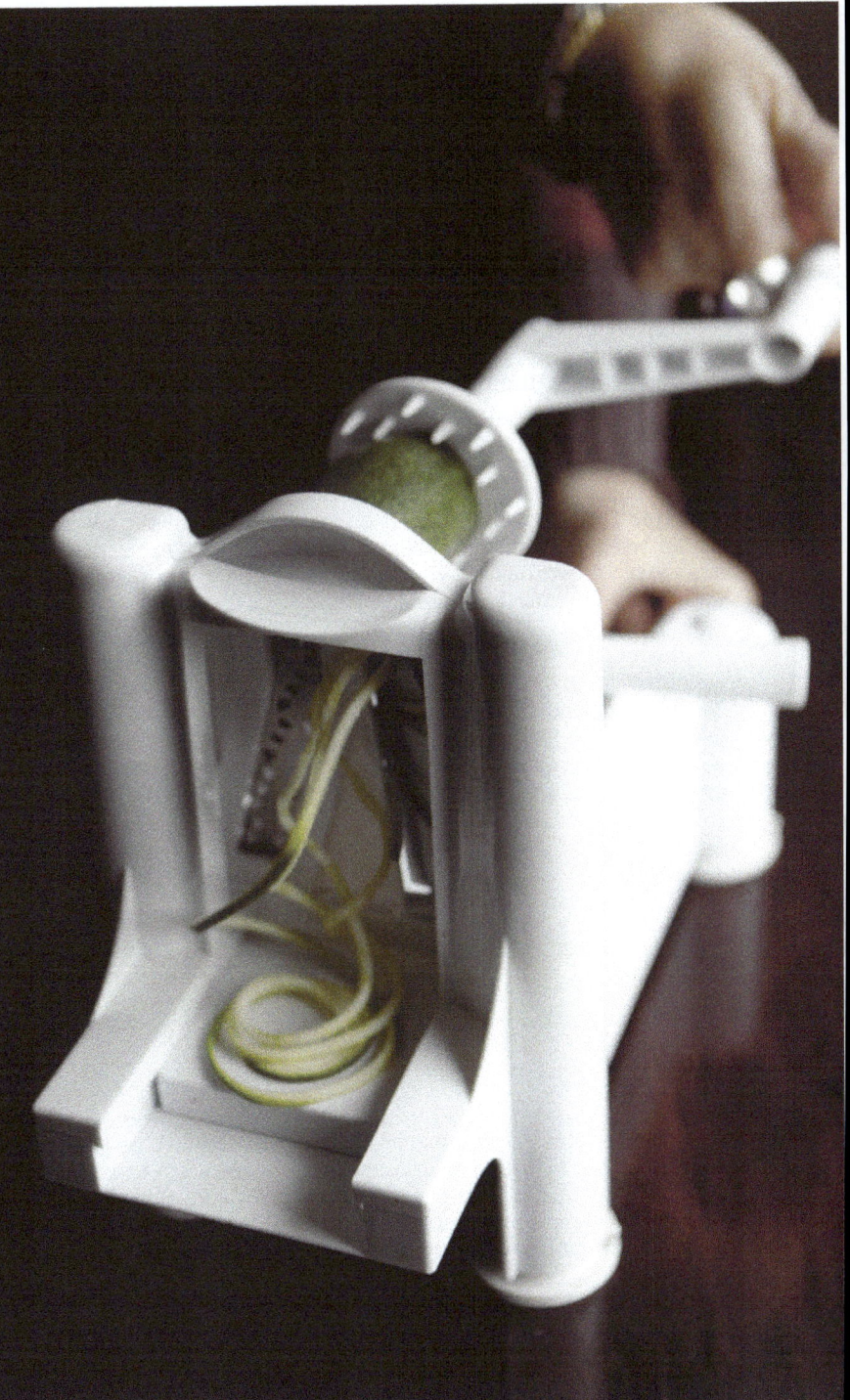

the power of sprouting ...

Sprouting is the 'germination' of a seed, nut or grain to increase and activate its enzymes and nutrient content. Sprouted foods differ from their original food source in a few key ways. Firstly, sprouting activates the enzymes and increases the vitamin and mineral content of the original food, especially the B vitamins. It can neutralize the substances in the plant which prevent the absorption of minerals. A good example of the difference between an original food and its sprouted counterpart are soybeans. Soybean sprouts contain up to 300% more Vitamin A and 500% more Vitamin C than its legume brother. The starches are converted into simple sugars making them much easier to digest. Another good example is sprouted wheat. It contains four times more niacin and twice as much folate and Vitamin B6 compared to whole wheat. Sprouts are lower in sugar and starch, making them ideal for diabetics, sugar addicts and anyone on a sugar-restricted diet. If you have poor absorption or digestive problems, sprouts would be the perfect addition to help increase your nutrient levels.

To sprout, it is important to soak the seeds, grains, nuts or legumes in water firstly, then place them in a bottle, jar or sprouter to grow. I have not included a huge amount of sprouted recipes within this book, as sprouting requires dedication and time which most people don't have. Any of the recipes within this book which contain nuts, seeds or grains can be replaced with the sprouted version of its original food. This is particularly useful for any raw food enthusiasts or those individuals who need extra nutrition with minimal digestion, for example, anyone fighting cancer or any individual with an inflammatory bowel condition like ulcerative colitis or Crohn's disease.

sprouting tips ...

Start with a clean organic seed, grain or nut and rinse thoroughly. Put the grain in a bowl or stainless steel pot and pour filtered water over the grain until it is covered. Let this soak for 5 to 6 hours or even overnight in water. In the morning, pour the grain through a sieve and rinse well. Spread the grain in a bottle, jar or sprouter and throughout the day continue to rinse the grain a few times. Continue rinsing the grains for two to three days until it has sprouted to your liking. When you are happy with the size of the sprouts, rinse and dry and put in the fridge until you are ready to eat.

SPROUTING CHART...

nut, seed or grain	soaking/sprouting	directions	nutrient potential
Adzuki beans	6 to 10hr / 2 to 5 days	Rinse and drain twice daily	Iron, niacin, calcium, lysine, A, C, E
Alfalfa – highly nutritious	8 to 12hr / 5 to 6 days	Rinse and drain twice daily	A, B, E, C, K, iron, calcium, potassium, zinc, chlorophyll, carotene, amino acids
Almonds – delicious. A soak, not a sprout.	8hr / Tail bulges, 2 days	Rinse twice daily every 8 hours	E, B2, B3, calcium, magnesium, phosphorous, manganese
Amaranth – a stubborn tiny sprout	None / 2 to 3 days	Rinse at least a few times daily	Calcium, iron, magnesium, potassium, selenium, B vitamins
Barley – not sweet – if left for too long it becomes a grass	6hr / 1 to 3 days	Rinse and drain twice daily	A, B2, magnesium, folate, potassium, lutein, zeaxanthin
Buckwheat (hulled groats)	1hr / 1 to 2 days	Rinse and drain twice daily	Phosphorous, folate, selenium, potassium, A, C, E, lecithin
Broccoli and radish sprouts	6 to 10 hr / 3 to 6 days	Rinse and drain twice daily	Broccoli – minerals, folate, C, A, K, lutein, zeaxanthin
Chickpeas	6 to 10hr / 2 to 5 days	Rinse and drain twice daily	Calcium, magnesium, phosphorous, folate, potassium, choline
Kamut – easy to grow	6 to 12hr / 2 to 3 days	Rinse and drain twice daily	C, E, B vitamins, magnesium, calcium
Lentils	7hr / 3 days	Rinse 2 to 3 times daily	Phosphorous, folate, potassium, Vitamin C, A, E iron, calcium
Millet – small and nutritious	6 to 10hr / 1 to 3 days	Rinse and drain every 8 to 12 hours	Vitamin B, C, E, iron, calcium, magnesium, B5, phosphorous

Item	Soak / Sprout Time	Rinsing	Nutrients
Mung Beans	6 to 10hr / 2 to 5 days	Rinse and drain twice daily	A, C, K, E, calcium, magnesium, iron, phosphorous, potassium
Oats – mildly sweet – quick to sprout	6hr / 1 to 3 days	Rinse and drain every 8 to 12 hours	A, B, C, E, phosphorous, potassium, iron
Pea	6 to 10hr / 2 to 5 days	Rinse and drain twice daily	A, C, B2, B3, B5, potassium, folate, manganese
Peanut	6 to 10hr / 2 to 5 days	Rinse and drain twice daily	A, B, C, E, calcium, iron, phosphorous,
Quinoa – super nutritious sprouts	1hr / 2 to 3 days	Rinse and drain every 8 to 12 hours	A, B, C, E, calcium, potassium, iron, phosphorous
Rice – short grain brown – bulging germ only	6 to 10hr / 2 to 3 days	Rinse and drain every 8 to 12 hours	B3, folate, potassium, phosphorous, magnesium
Rye – sweet and nutritious	8hr / 2 to 3 days	Rinse and drain every 8 to 12 hours	B, C, E, calcium, iron, phosphorous
Sesame – fast, small, nutritious	2 to 8hr / 1 to 3 days	Rinse and drain every 8 to 12 hours	B, C, E, calcium, iron, magnesium
Spelt – very nutritious	6 to 12hr / 2 to 3 days	Rinse and drain every 8 to 12 hours	A, B, C, E, K, chlorophyll, iron, lecithin, calcium, B5
Sunflower – a soak, not sprout	1hr / Done in 12hr	None	B complex, calcium, iron, phosphorous
Tritacle – nutritious – a combination of wheat and rye	6 to 8hr / 2 to 3 days	Rinse and drain every 8 to 12 hours	B complex, C, E and many minerals
Wheat Berries – sweet and nutritious	6 to 12hr / 2 to 3 days	Rinse and drain every 8 to 12 hours	B Complex, C, E, magnesium, phosphorous, folate
Wild Rice	9hr / 3 to 5 days	Rinse and drain every 8 to 12 hours	B complex
All other nuts	6hr / No sprouting – just soaking	This will soften then for dishes.	Rich in protein, B complex, fibre and minerals

shopping checklist ...

The following ingredients are the foods, herbs and spices that I use in my raw food kitchen. Most of these foods are available at the supermarket, local health food stores or farmer markets. You may not be familiar with some of these ingredients, which is why I love to describe what they are and their important roles in restoring health.

FRESH HERBS and SPICES ...

I always have fresh herbs on hand to add flavour and nutrition to my living food recipes. Herbs are packed full of minerals, vitamins and phytochemicals that not only add taste and flavor, but some incredible healing potential. Some of my favourite herbs include:

Ginger is great to throw in dishes if you want to relieve nausea, queasiness, gas or heartburn. It boosts blood circulation, reduces inflammation linked to PMS and headaches and helps to prevent ovarian and colorectal cancer. No wonder I add this zesty herb to most of my raw creations.

Garlic is a natural antibiotic that can wipe out hundreds of nasty bacterial, fungal and viral infections. It is nature's strongest weapon in the fight against disease as it can provide amazing defenses against all types of cancer. It is a heart loving herb that can lower high blood pressure, cholesterol and guard against dangerous blood clots.

Onions provide great cardiovascular and cancer protecting qualities. They encourage the growth of 'friendly bacteria' in the small intestines to protect against tummy bugs and gastrointestinal cancers. If you want to improve your respiratory system, don't forget to add a fresh onion to your dish. It is one of the best foods to remove mucous off the chest.

Jalapeno peppers will put some fire into your blood, which is great for anyone with poor circulation, cold hands or chilblains. This little chilli pepper is brilliant for clearing congestion, boosting energy and burning away stubborn fat. You can also add this herb to clear headaches, prevent blood clotting or to reduce inflammation linked to arthritis, psoriasis and nerve damage.

Coriander is a wonderful anti-diabetic herb that stimulates insulin to lower blood sugar. It protects against atherosclerosis by reducing the 'bad' cholesterol and eases diarrhea caused from nasty bacteria and fungus. The natural oils found in coriander help to heal mouth ulcers while freshening the breath. It is an iron rich herb that prevents anemia and one of the best herbs for removing heavy metals like aluminium, lead and mercury from the body.

Depending on which dishes I am cooking I also like to have on hand:

Basil was revered in ancient times for its medicinal qualities. Fresh basil contains the pungent oils, camphor and thymol. These anti-bacterial and anti-viral oils can wipe out bronchitis, sinusitis, colds and even staphylococcus bacteria.

It has some beautiful anti-inflammatory properties that can ease arthritis and inflammatory bowel problems. In Scotland it is known as the 'herb of gladness' as it lifts the dark cloud of depression while easing stress and tension.

Mint is an old folk remedy for bad breath and digestive problems. It eases irritable bowel, upset tummies and nausea. It contains perillyl alcohol, a substance which protects against colon, skin and lung cancer. If you are suffering from nausea or headaches, mint is brilliant to add to dishes. The natural menthol found in mint can clear congestion in the nose, throat and lungs.

Parsley is one of the best sources of Vitamin A, C and chlorophyll. A high intake of these vitamins can prevent diabetes, cardiovascular disease and cancer. It is a natural diuretic that reduces fluid retention, gravel, stones and urinary problems. If your joints are stiff or your knuckles are swollen, add some fresh parsley to remedy this. For colic, indigestion and an unsettled stomach parsley works wonders. The essential oils found in parsley are one of the best remedies for cellulite.

Dill is the perfect digestive tonic as it helps to keep the bowels regular while relieving diarrhea caused from microbes, fungus or bacteria. No wonder Indians often use dill in yoghurt, as this little herb is the perfect remedy for dysentery. If you are suffering from hiccups chew on dill seeds or leaves – their calming nature can expel gas. Dill calms frazzled nerves and sleeplessness. Like fennel, dill can stimulate milk flow in nursing mothers.

Fennel is the perfect herb to overcome anemia, because of its rich iron content. In India, fennel seeds are chewed to relieve indigestion and a nasty case of 'bad breath'. They are great for stomach spasms, irritable bowel, gas, bloating and constipation. Fennel can be used by pregnant mothers to increase the quality and quantity of milk. It is often made into a tea and used as an eye wash for conjunctivitis and other eye inflammations. It is a perfect remedy for children.

DRIED HERBS and SPICES ...

Fresh herbs are definitely the highest in nutritional value. Dried herbs are the next best option if you do not have access to organic, fresh herbs. They last for ages and I keep these in glass jars in the cupboard. Look for organic herbs to ensure they are not laced with pesticides. The best herbs to have on hand are:

Black Peppercorns were used in ancient times by the Romans to pay taxes, instead of coins. Black peppercorns have been revered for 4000 years and were used to ease muscle aches, pains, arthritis and stiffness. I also like to use green peppercorns in my dishes.

Cayenne arrived in the West from India in 1548. This hot red chilli contains capsaicin, a powerful stimulant and immune boosting ingredient. It guards against prostate cancer, rebuilds blood health, removes toxins and prevents heart attacks. Its heating qualities can boost circulation, enhance metabolism and weight loss and lower cholesterol. The healing qualities of cayenne are endless and lots of information can be found about this wonder spice throughout the book.

Cinnamon is an old spice that originated in Sri Lanka. It is revered by the Chinese as a 'cure all' and used in Ayruvedic remedies to relieve upset tummies, indigestion, nausea, vomiting and colic. It is great remedy for diarrhea and blood blood sugar problems. If you suffer from candida, cinnamon is the spice to wipe out this virulent fungus. The essential oils in cinnamon can relieve exhaustion, depression and weakness.

Cumin contains good amounts of iron to boost immunity and to improve oxygen levels in the blood. New studies are highlighting its benefit in protecting against liver and stomach tumours. It is a great spice to enhance liver detoxification and has been well known throughout history for its digestion healing properties.

Curry leaves were used by traditional practitioners to stop greying of the hair. They are added to dishes in the orient to kill microbes that cause diarrhea, dysentery and stomach bugs. No wonder curry is the main dish served in Asian countries. New studies are proving that curry leaves are a great anti-diabetic herb, as well as a powerful herb to prevent skin and stomach cancer.

Lime leaves are brilliant for preventing and treating colds, sore throats, coughs and fevers. They are natural calming agents that can ease a bad case of frazzled nerves or anxiety. Kaffir lime leaves are great for healing the gums and any digestive upset.

Mustard seeds boost blood circulation and in doing so, help to ease muscle pain, neuralgia and spasms. They quell a nasty fever and fight colds and flu's. If your bowels are sluggish or you feel nauseous, add some mustard seeds to your next dish.

Nutmeg has been used by the Chinese since the 7th Century as a tonic for stomach problems. It is one of the best remedies for stomach cramps, nausea, diarrhea, flatulence and vomiting.

Oregano is a warming herb that clears congestion, coughs and respiratory ailments. It can kill bacteria, fungi and worms and the oil is a brilliant remedy for head lice in children.

Paprika is made from sweet red chilli's or chilli peppers. Like its brother cayenne, it contains capsaicin, a very strong antioxidant and anti-inflammatory that can guard against cancer and cardiovascular disease.

Rosemary was found in the first Dynasty tombs of the ancient Egyptians. It was revered for its ability to improve memory and protect the brain against ageing and damage. It is brilliant for stress, depression, exhaustion and tension. The oil can encourage hair growth and restore lost hair colour.

Thyme was used by the Egyptians to embalm royalty and given to soldiers to evoke courage before going into battle. Today it is used to relieve spasmodic coughing, bronchitis, catarrh and asthma. It boosts immunity and fights all types of bacterial infections.

Turmeric is the most powerful anti-cancer herb found on the planet. It contains vast amounts of curcuminoids, powerful substances that have shown to halt all phases of cancer. The health properties of turmeric are endless. More information about this wonder herb can be found throughout the book.

Vanilla pods/beans were used by the Mayans to flavour chocolate drinks centuries before the Spanish entered Mexico in 1542. Vanilla pods contain countless minerals, phytonutrients, essential oils and vitamins. Vanilla is a powerful aphrodisiac that can treat many different sexual problems. This sensuous spice has both uplifting and calming properties. It eases depression, anger, irritability and even sleeping problems. I often use real vanilla beans or pods in my dishes. If you want a quicker option, look for pure vanilla essence or extract made from the whole vanilla pods, without the alcohol. The seeds from 1 vanilla bean equals around 1 tablespoon of vanilla extract. To de-seed a vanilla bean, cut it long ways, open up and run the spoon along the edge to catch the seeds and oil. This is what you will use in the recipe. You can also use the pod if you don't mind a bit of crunch.

Wasabi – When we think of wasabi, most of us think of the green paste that we eat with sushi in Japanese restaurants. This is not actually wasabi, it is horseradish, mixed with mustard and food colouring. True wasabi is wasabi japonica, a root vegetable and relative of the watercress family. It is ground into a paste and served in Japanese dishes. It contains the same detoxifying substances found in broccoli that help to stop cancer-causing agents from invoking cancer. True wasabi is an anti-inflammatory and anti-clotting agent that can reduce the risk of heart disease and strokes. To get the benefits of wasabi, make sure it is wasabi paste you are buying. Otherwise, look for pure horseradish paste. Horseradish is brilliant for sinusitis and any other form of mucous congestion.

NUTS and SEEDS ...

Raw nuts and seeds are the prime base for most recipes in a 'living food' kitchen. Most nuts keep for many months if bought fresh and stored well. I store my nuts in glass jars in the fridge to prevent rancidity. Ideally nuts and seeds should be soaked overnight and rinsed well before use. Personally I don't always have time to soak my nuts and seeds for this amount of time and you may find me eating un-soaked nuts. These will also work well in any of my dishes. Nuts and seeds are loaded with protein, minerals, vitamins, natural oils and antioxidants to fight wrinkles and to reduce the risk of heart disease, cancer and diabetes. They are brilliant for maintaining a fast metabolism. My favourites include:

Almond
Brazil nut
Cashew
Chia seeds
Coconut, dried and shredded
Flaxseeds or Flaxseed meal
Hazelnut
Macadamia
Pecan – great for bases in raw desserts
Pine Nut
Pistachio
Pumpkin seed
Sesame seed (white and black)
Sunflower seed
Walnut

NUT and SEED BUTTERS ...

If you have nuts and seeds at home and a good food processor, then you can turn any nut and seed into delicious nut butters. They are also handy to keep in the cupboard for many different dishes. More information about nuts and seeds can be found in special drinks.

Almond Butter is made from pressed almonds. It is low in saturated fats and high in healthy monounsaturated fats to lower cholesterol and protect the heart. It contains huge amounts of protein, calcium, fibre, magnesium, folic acid, potassium, beta-sitosterol and Vitamin E.

Cashew Butter is high in protein, low in saturated fats and rich in healthy monounsaturated fats to reduce cholesterol and stabilize blood sugar. It contains good amounts of copper for healthy blood and magnesium for bone, nerve and muscle strengthening qualities.

Hazelnut Butter is a delicious heart smart butter. It contains healthy oleic acid to lower cholesterol and plenty of calcium, magnesium and potassium to lower blood pressure. Its high arginine content helps to relax blood vessels giving protection against breast cancer. It also contain good amounts of protein, B vitamins, E, iron, zinc and phytosterols and folate, flavonoids and anthocyanidins to decrease the risk of cancer, heart disease and depression.

Tahini is made from sesame seeds. You can get white tahini (made from white sesame seeds) and black tahini (made from black sesame seeds). You can also get hulled tahini (removal of the husks – either with chemicals or mechanically) or unhulled (where the husks are left in place). Unhulled tahini contains larger amounts of calcium, but it is calcium oxalate, which is not considered highly absorbable.

Cacao or cocoa butter is the cream coloured fat extracted from cacao seeds (cocoa beans) used to flavour and add smoothness to chocolate, tanning oils and other foods. It contains high amounts of magnesium to help with PMS, headaches and muscle cramps. Cocoa butter, found in dark chocolate contains oleic acid to lower LDL cholesterol and raise HDL cholesterol (the good fat). Cocoa butter is brilliant for raising serotonin and endorphins in the brain to uplift moods. No wonder chocolate is often coined the 'love drug'.

NATURAL SWEETENERS ...

In 'Raw Addiction' I use lots of natural fruits, like medjool dates to sweeten dishes. If the recipe needs a creamier texture, then raw honey, agave or yacon syrup can be used. I have listed a number of 'natural sugar alternatives' below which are not in many of my recipes, but can be substituted for anyone on a sugar free, low glycemic diet, like those fighting cancer, obesity or diabetes. Some alternatives are better than others, and great natural sugar swap alternatives can be found in the chapter 'Sweet Treats'. For those who have a sweet tooth, but do not want to feel guilty about over-indulging in too much sugar, then the healthier sugar options are below:

Ripe fresh fruits contain the complete package for ideal health just as nature intended it - nutrients, fibre, water and fruit sugars. The ripest fruits grown without chemicals are the sweetest and they are definitely the best for sweetening dishes. I often let my bananas and mangoes ripen, I peel them and place in the freezer. These taste great in green smoothies, raw cakes, mousses and other dishes.

Dried Fruits are perfect for flavouring cereals, smoothies and desserts. If you need a syrup consistency, soak them in water and blend to prepare the dish. Dates, figs and prunes are fantastic for this. If you buy dried fruits, look for naturally dried fruits free from sulfur dioxide. To ensure you are getting 'raw' why not try dehydrating yourself.

Dates are one of my favourite natural sweeteners. Even though they rate a little higher on the glycemic index, you only need to use small amounts of these to sweeten dishes (which rates them lower in sugar anyway). Medjool dates supply huge amounts of fibre to lower cholesterol and prevent colon and breast cancer. They contain flavonoids, beta-carotene, lutein and zeaxanthin. These are powerful antioxidants that protect cells against free radical damage, as well as guard against prostate, breast, lung, endometrial and pancreatic cancer. Dates are a very good source of iron to prevent anemia and boost hemoglobin levels (oxygen carrying molecule in red blood cells). On top of this, they contain potassium, copper, calcium, manganese and magnesium to fortify the blood and protect the bones, teeth, nerves and muscles. Dates also contain good amounts of B vitamins to boost energy levels. So even though their fructose content is a little higher than most fruits, their healing potential far outweighs any disadvantage of this.

Goji berries are known as the 'fruit of longevity' in China. They are rich in germanium, an amazing substance that oxygenates the body's cells. Goji also contains skin protecting phytochemicals and an abundant array of 19 amino acids, 21 minerals, essential fatty acids, beta-sitosterol (prostate cancer protection) and countless other cancer-fighting antioxidants. This little berry contains more Vitamin C than an orange and more iron than a steak. Traditional healers used goji berries to enhance fertility, virility and immunity. Always purchase a highly reputable source of naturally dried organic goji berries to ensure they haven't been stored for long periods of time. I love goji berries, I just wish I could eat them fresh off trees.

Lucuma is an amazing Peruvian fruit with an exotic taste and smell. It has a similar taste to maple syrup and is brilliant to use in chocolate or vanilla desserts. It is a good source of natural carbohydrates, fibre, vitamins and minerals including beta-carotene, Vitamin B3 and iron. The Peruvian's call this fruit the 'Gold of the Incas' as it was considered one of their finest medicinal tonics. Lucuma has anti-inflammatory qualities that can improve wound healing and prevent skin ageing. Even though this fruit tastes sweet, it does not increase your blood sugar unlike other sweeteners, making it a good alternative to sugar.

Mesquite powder is taken from the pods of the native South American mesquite tree. It is then ground into a flour and adds a sweet, malty or carob like flavour to recipes. It is very good at balancing blood sugar levels. The flour is an excellent form of fibre, meeting daily needs in just 2 tablespoons. It contains good amounts of lysine as well as protein, calcium, magnesium, potassium, iron and zinc. The ancient Native Americans relied on mesquite as a staple food. Mesquite works well with both vanilla and chocolate dishes and is a great addition to smoothies or natural ice-cream.

Agave syrup is derived from the agave plant. It is important to be careful with buying this syrup, as even if it says it is raw, it may not be. To make agave syrup/nectar, the plant needs to be heated at temperatures above 140 F for 36 hours to develop its sweetness and to turn it into a syrup. The main carbohydrates in agave are complex forms of fructose known as fructosans. When heated these fructosan units are broken down into fructose units, then filtered. So to get agave from the plant it needs to be boiled, then filtered, which can leave the syrup lacking in vital nutrients found in the original plant. Even though it is claimed to be 'low glycemic' it still contains a concentration of 90% fructose to 10% glucose. Fructose in large amounts can raise glucose levels. Don't get me wrong, it is definitely a far better alternative to sugar and other sugar substitutes, but like any other natural sweetener it should still be used moderately in pure, raw, organic form.

Maple syrup is not a raw food, but it tastes great and has some nutritional value. It contains good amounts of manganese to nourish nerves, antioxidant defenses and energy production. It also supplies fair amounts of zinc to help boost white blood cell defenses against colds, flu's and viruses. Look for grade B maple syrup for a higher vitamin and mineral content. Once again, it is a little higher in glycemic index, so use moderately, but it is definitely a worthy substitute over refined sugar.

Honey, when raw and unprocessed is a 'super food' that contains countless antioxidants, minerals, vitamins, enzymes and natural antibiotics to boost immunity and guard against viruses and microbes. However, processed honey (commonly found in supermarkets) is stripped of these nutrients and is no better than common table sugar. The beauty of honey is, even though it is sweet, it contains large amounts of healing nutrients. Just like agave and maple syrup, honey should still be used moderately. I always get my honey straight from the bees.

Xylitol is a natural sugar alcohol that is found in certain fruits and vegetables. It has been used since the 1940's to prevent tooth decay and is found in many chewing gums. It contains 45% less calories than sugar and 75% less carbohydrates. The original source of xylitol was Scandinavian birch trees, but due to their rarity now, true xylitol is hard to find and quite expensive. China and Asia are now extracting xylitol from corn husks – which cannot compare to the original birch source. If you cannot find pure birch tree xylitol, I would seek out xylitol made from organic corn. The glycemic index of xylitol is only 7. Some people do get mild tummy upsets from this product.

Stevia is an amazing herb that I have been using for over fifteen years. It is 300 times sweeter than sucrose, yet rates at zero on a glycemic index and has next to no calories. It does not cause spikes in blood sugar, making it a popular alternative amongst diabetics. The problem with stevia is even though it is sweet, it is slightly bitter in taste. I love the bitterness of stevia and it is a superb natural sweetener for anyone on sugar-restricted diets. If you cannot get fresh leaves, you can buy the whole leaf powder. It is hard to find a stevia liquid that hasn't been highly processed, but if you can find a pure stevia extract that hasn't been subjected to high heats, you will be amazed at how beautifully sweetens dishes.

Lo Han Guo / Kuo is a natural sweetener taken from the fruit of the 'siraitia grosvenoril' plant, a native of China and Northern Thailand. It contains no calories or glycemic index, yet has been used for thousands of years for its medicinal properties. In China this fruit is known as the fruit of 'longevity' and in fact the locals who cultivate this plant have a large number of centurians among their people. The sweetness of this fruit comes from the triterpene glycoside compounds which are called mogrosides. These compounds make up 1% of the fruit, they are extracted into a powder which is 80% mogrosides. Be dubious when looking for a good source of this fruit, most companies combine a small amount of the fruit with fructose or maltodextrin from corn and call it Lo Han Guo.

Erythritol are natural 'sugar alcohols' found in fruits and vegetables like melons, pears, mushrooms and fermented foods. It is made from plant sugars that are mixed with water and then fermented with a natural culture, turning it into erythritol. It is then filtered, crystallized then dried. It looks like sugar and doesn't have the bitter taste of stevia. It is considered one of the healthiest, safest and lowest calorie sugar alternatives to use as a natural sweetener as it contains no calories or glycemic index. Sometimes stevia and xylitol can cause diarrhea or stomach upsets in some people, whereas erythritol rarely does this. Like xylitol, it does not cause tooth decay.

Yacon syrup is extracted from the yacon plant, a native plant grown throughout Coloumbia, Peru, Ecuador and Bolivia. It is a brilliant source of iron and a natural pre-biotic that can improve digestive and colon function. It is recommended for diabetics as it contains half the calories of honey and is much lower in glycemic index than most natural sweeteners, running at 1. It is a heart-loving sweetener that can thin blood, lower blood pressure and cholesterol and prevent blood clotting. It is a rich source of fructooligosacchardes (FOS), a dietary sugar that helps with weight management and prevention of chronic diseases like cancer. It does not cause spikes in blood sugar due to of its high levels of FOS making it a perfect choice for raw food enthusiasts to sweeten dishes. To ensure it stays raw, it must be produced at temperatures below 40 degrees C. This is one of my favourite sweeteners largely due to its immense healing properties.

SALTS...

Common table salt is dangerous. It is refined and 82 of the 84 minerals are removed leaving only sodium and chloride. An excessive intake of chloride causes hypertension, liver, kidney and heart problems and adrenal exhaustion. Common salt was also de-iodized (removal of iodine) resulting in thyroid problems, fibrocystic breasts and even cancer. Normal sea salt is salt taken from the ocean, yet it is normally refined at high temperatures leaving it with little enzyme or mineral content.

Celtic Salt would have to be my favourite natural salt alternative. It is a naturally moist, salt taken from the Atlantic seawater off the coast of Brittany, France. It is harvested using the traditional Celtic method of wooden rakes. It is air and sun dried in clay ponds and gathered with wooden tools to preserve the minerals and enzymes. Because it is not refined, it contains all 84 live elements, like those found in sea water. Celtic salt contains potassium, iodine, zinc and magnesium to ensure that any unused sodium is excreted harmlessly via the kidneys. Celtic salt helps to nourish the body with minerals. I often use this in water to help clear sinuses or bronchial congestion and it works brilliantly in a bath to relieve muscle aches and pains. Its rich alkaline mineral content ensures that the body is able to remove acidity. These are only some of the healing effects of celtic salt and as you can see by my recipes it is always my favourite salt addition.

Himalayan Crystal Salt originates from the Khewra salt mines in Pakistan, located 300 km from the Himalaya. It is claimed to contain all 84 minerals, just like celtic salt and producers proclaim that it can help with fluid retention, respiratory problems, mucous build-up, vascular health, blood sugar imbalance and other problems. In 2003, 15 specimens of Himalaya rock salt were analysed by the Bavarian Protection agency. They found that there was a large variation of minerals in all of the specimens. Be very careful when purchasing Himalayan salt, as some dubious Pakistan companies package cheap 'rock salt' and sell this as 'himalayan salt'. There is also some suspicion that the fluoride and heavy metal content in some brands of this salt is very high. Look for a reputable source.

Tamari is a type of soy sauce that is made from the fermentation of soybeans, water and sea salt. It is much lower in sodium than soy sauce and contains some useful nutrients, compared to its processed counterpart soy sauce. Tamari is rich in tryptophan, manganese, Vitamin B3 and protein. Tryptophan is needed to make serotonin, a neurotransmitter that helps with sleep and stable moods. I love tamari and I use it in most dishes. Always look for naturally fermented, organic, wheat free tamari.

Braggs Amino Acid Seasoning is a liquid protein concentrate, derived from GMO free soybeans. It contains all 16 amino acids, both essential and non-essential, making it a superb protein source for vegetarians. Bragg's has a very savoury, 'meaty' full bodied flavour and can be used interchangeably between tamari and celtic salt. Fermented soy products have been linked to a lower risk of breast, prostate and colon cancer. Soy protein also helps to reduce menopausal symptoms and osteoporosis.

Miso is a fermented soybean paste that is made using cooked soybeans, koji, salt and sometimes different grains like rice or barley. There are a number of different types of miso all with different health promoting properties. I use miso in a lot of different dishes – it is rich in Vitamin B12 and alkaline in nature, making it a natural detoxifying food. Always buy unpasteurized miso as it is a 'living food'. Use moderately if you have candida or a fungal problem.

OILS ...

When purchasing oils always buy organic, GMO free, unrefined oils found in dark bottles, that have not been exposed to heat, sunlight or contamination. It is important to make sure that the oil is processed quickly after harvesting. To find out more about the healing properties of different oils, refer to 'salad dressings'.

Olive oil contains all of the healing properties of olives (listed below), plus huge amounts of monounsaturated fats to lower cholesterol and protect the heart. When buying olive oil, purchase organic, extra virgin, first cold pressed olive oil to ensure you receive all of the Vitamin E, polyphenols and healthy fats from this magical oil.

Flaxseed oil is one of the best sources of omega 3 fatty acids in the world. Omega 3 fats prevent inflammation linked to heart disease, PMS, arthritis, psoriasis, eczema, autoimmune conditions and more. Be careful when buying flaxseed oil, as flaxseeds go rancid quickly after picking. Always question the source of your flaxseeds and make sure the oil has been extracted on harvesting.

Hemp Seed oil is the 'master of oils' as it contains a perfect balance of omega 3, 6 and 9 oils. Fifteen years ago I discovered this oil while visiting a 'natural products expo' in America and I have never looked back. It contains all essential and non-essential amino acids as well as plenty of vitamins, minerals and antioxidants.

Udo's oil has been another favourite of mine for many years. After only a few days of using this, my hair becomes stronger and shinier and my skin takes on a velvety glow. It contains a good balance of omega 3, 6 and 9 and is made from organic, GMO free flaxseeds, sunflower, sesame, rice and oat germs, coconut, evening primrose, rosemary, lecithin and Vitamin E. I love this oil - it makes your hair, skin and nails strong, luscious and youthful.

Coconut oil, found in a raw and unrefined state contains a unique saturated fat known as lauric acid. Lauric acid helps to speed up weight loss and boost immunity while killing nasty parasites, bacteria and fungi. It is brilliant to use in desserts, raw food sweet treats and other Asian inspired dishes.

Sesame oil is a very healthy oil, low in saturated fats and high in healthy monounsaturated and polyunsaturated fats. It is a heart loving oil that can lower cholesterol and blood pressure. Ayurvedic practitioners have used this for four thousand years to treat burns, psoriasis, skin infections and toxicity problems. This is my favourite oil to use in Asian salad dressings and noodle dishes.

OLIVES ...

Olives are full of healing phytonutrients. One of these is hydroxytryosol, a substance which prevents cancer and osteoporosis. Olives can block histamine receptors making them a great anti-allergy fruit. They are loaded with healthy fats like oleic acid. This fat reduces cholesterol and cardiovascular disease. In terms of nutrient content, this fruit is nothing short of astounding. They contain huge amounts of Vitamin E, zinc and selenium to fend off disease. No wonder the Mediterranean people have such low levels of cancer and cardiovascular disease. Did you know that all olives begin green? They start out green and it is during the ripening or curing process that they darken. This depends on the method which is used to cure the olive – water, soaking in oil, brine or dry packing in salt. The most artificial method of curing is soaking the olives in lye, which removes the bitterness, flavour and healing properties. Lye is a poison – basically it is caustic soda, the same thing that is used to clean drainpipes. To avoid the consumption of drainpipe chemicals do not eat lye cured olives. Seek out naturally cured olives.

VINEGARS ...

Vinegar is made by the result of harmless micro-organisms (yeast and 'acetobacter') that turn sugars into acetic acid. Many healthy foods like yoghurt, cheese, apple cider vinegar and miso involve some type of bacteria in their production. The first process is known as alcoholic fermentation and it occurs when yeasts change natural sugars to alcohol. In the second process, a group of bacteria converts the alcohol portion to acid. This is the acetic acid fermentation that forms vinegar. Vinegar contains many vitamins and compounds like Vitamin B1, B2 and mineral salts. Its nutrient content is highly dependent on the original substance that was used to make the vinegar. Always buy undistilled, raw vinegar that has not been exposed to heat.

Apple Cider Vinegar is a wonderful source of malic acid, a substance which aids protein digestion and boosts immunity. It is also a good source of potassium, sodium, phosphorous, sulpher, copper, silica and other trace minerals to enhance all aspects of health. When buying apple cider vinegar it should be unfiltered, unpasteurized and made from the whole organic apples and contain the 'mother' for nutritional purposes.

Balsamic Vinegar has been made for thousands of years in northern Italy. This vinegar is made from the reduced juice of sweet white grapes like the Trebbiano or Lambrusco varieties and aged for 12 years or more in wooden casks. Most balsamic vinegars are processed quickly and therefore lose most of their nutritional value. Look for a high quality balsamic vinegar that has aged for a number of years in wooden casks to ensure you receive its healing qualities.

Rice Vinegar has been made in China and Japan for thousands of years from rice wine or sake. It comes in three varieties, white, red or black – all with varying medicinal properties. On the island of Kyushu in southern Japan, a black variety of rice vinegar is made from thick brown rice sake. This vinegar is sweet and holds some great medicinal properties. Rice vinegar is excellent for killing bacteria on foods. I use brown rice vinegar in my dishes – it is made from organic brown rice, well water and seed vinegar and procured over six to ten months in vats. It contains many healthy enzymes to improve digestion.

WHOLEGRAINS and LEGUMES ...

Most of the wholegrains and legumes that I use in 'Raw Addiction' are soaked or sprouted to release their healing potential. I have only listed the whole grains that I consume most commonly in these dishes. Please feel free to add these healthy grains to any dishes to increase your satiety and healing value.

Quinoa is a relative of amaranth. It is known as the 'mother grain' as it has the highest protein content of all the grains. It digests very slowly, making it superb for weight loss. It contains good amounts of B vitamins and folate for healthy nerves and loads of calcium to strengthen bones and teeth.

Amaranth is another protein enriched grain that is brimming with minerals like iron, calcium and manganese and vitamins like C, A, K, B6 and folate. It is one of the best sources of lysine to prevent herpes and cancer.

Barley is a nourishing grain that is beneficial during convalescence. I would not incorporate this as a prime grain to fight cancer, but barley soup can be used to build strength following surgery or if sick during chemotherapy. This ancient grain contains soluble fibre to metabolise fats and carbohydrates and to lower cholesterol and insoluble fibre to remove toxins from the digestive tract that can cause colon cancer. Barley contains good amounts of niacin to protect the heart and high amounts of vitamin E to thin the blood.

Brown Rice is a rich source of B vitamins to boost energy and calm the nerves. It is useful following orthodox cancer treatments, when energy levels are low or nerves are frazzled. One cup of brown rice supplies 88% of the RDA of manganese. Manganese is a part of a powerful enzyme known as superoxide dismutase (SOD). SOD guards against free radical damage that causes cancer. People who regularly consume brown rice are less likely to gain weight and suffer from diabetes, heart disease or strokes.

Buckwheat is a beautiful alkalizing grain that improves the appetite and helps to quell diarrhea. It contains good amounts of rutin to give protection against radiation and x-rays. Buckwheat sprouts are a brilliant source of chlorophyll, enzymes and vitamins.

Millet is an alkaline grain and one of the best grains used in cancer therapy. It has a very rich amino acid profile and is a good source of silica to beautify hair, skin and nails. Millet can prevent constipation and is a good remedy for migraines.

SEAWEEDS ...

Seaweeds bathe in mineral rich oceans and because of this they absorb huge amounts of minerals like calcium, magnesium, zinc and iodine, which are then passed onto you when you eat the seaweed. Hijike, arame, kombu and wakame are known as 'brown algae'. They are brilliant for detoxifying heavy metals and radiation from the body. All seaweeds improve hair health and growth and enhance beautiful skin and metabolic function. Their rich iodine content helps to guard against thyroid problems, fibrocystic breast disease, weight gain and breast cancer. Dulse is a red seaweed that is prevalent in arctic waters. It contains up to 112 minerals and healing elements, including up to 34 times the potassium content of a banana. It contains high amounts of the omega 3 fats, EPA and DHA and the highest polyphenol content of any seaweed, giving it amazing cancer inhibiting properties. I love seaweeds – when buying these look for a reputable source to ensure the seaweeds you are eating haven't been tainted with toxins or heavy metals. Try out the yummy Red Dulse Salad with a lime infusion in 'Raw Addiction'.

CHOCOLATE SWEETENERS ...

Cacao Beans, Nibs and Powder are obtained from the cacao theobroma plant and are the source of all chocolate and cocoa products. Theobroma translates to the 'food of the gods' and the Mexican named this prized seed 'chocolate'. Cacao contains more antioxidant flavonoids than any other food including green tea and blueberries. Calcium, zinc, iron, copper, sulfur, potassium, proteins, magnesium, beta-carotene, lipase, lysine and other powerful substances are found in this amazing powder.

Cocoa Powder is made from dried, fermented cocoa beans. When made naturally, it is full of antioxidants and protein, just like its brother cacao. However, it is important to beware of cheap, highly processed imitations.

Carob obtained its name from the carob pod of a tree that is native to the Mediterranean. It has been used by the Greeks for four thousand years to sweeten dishes and for its medicinal properties. It contains plenty of natural sugars and is useful for treating diarrhea and high cholesterol. It contains theobromine, so it should be used cautiously in anyone with hypersensitivity problems.

how to use this book ...

As I have mentioned previously, this book is great for everyone. Originally I planned to include symbols to indicate if a recipe was gluten free, wheat free, sugar free and so on and then I realised that nearly every recipe within this book is allergen free in some way. 'Raw Addiction' is the perfect healthy eating guide for anyone with food intolerances or allergies. Some of the recipes contain nuts and fermented soy products, so if you are sensitive to these, simply leave them out of the recipes or swap for a non-allergenic alternative.

Personally I do not like a lot of gluten free products as they are often bland and lacking in nutrition. The gluten-free recipes found within 'Raw Addiction' are nutritious and absolutely delicious. On top of this, all of the recipes are dairy and animal product free, making this a perfect book for vegans and vegetarians.

If you are a busy person like me, you probably don't have a lot of spare time to spend in the kitchen preparing food. Because of this reason I now use a lot of shortcuts, like using easier ingredients to speed up my prep time - if you don't have time to soak nuts and seeds, simply throw in fresh. Please feel free to alter or adapt any of my recipes to suit your needs and time frame.

If you are on a completely sugar-free diet, like diabetics or anyone fighting cancer, I would swap maple syrup, agave or honey in the recipes for pure forms of stevia, erythritol, pure birch xylitol, medjool dates or yacon syrup. To further increase the nutritional impact of these recipes, why not try replacing any of the nuts, seeds or grains for their sprouted counterparts, to increase their healing value even more. If you feel you cannot go completely raw, that's okay, just start slowly and use the salads and recipes found in this book to go with your cooked forms of protein like quinoa, brown rice, fish, eggs or others.

Every recipe within this book is focused not only on raw and living eco-conscious selections, but also on nutritional impact, balance and healing quality. When creating these dishes, I was looking to blend incredible flavors and textures, whilst creating healing dishes balanced synergistically with the right vitamins, minerals, amino acids, omega oils and antioxidants. Each recipe is designed to not only be delicious, but to powerfully enhance & transform your health, on every level.

Nutty Milks
Nutty Almond Milk
Vanilla Hazelnut Swirl
Berry Mocha
Hazelnut Cinnamon
Chocaholic

Super Fruit Smoothies
Mango Tango
Dance in the Tropics
Immune Booster
Melon Madness
Pine-Lime Punch

Green Smoothie Madness
Super Green
Digestive-Ease
Go for Gold
Supermodel Skin
For the Love of Green
Tropical Antioxidant
Number #1 Green Smoothie
Bathroom Bliss

'Shake It Up' Power Drinks
Goji Heaven
Cancer-Kicking Power Shake
Chocolate Rocket Fuel

Juices
Heavy Metal Detox
Super 9
Resveratrol Treat
Anti-Cancer Vitamin Pill
Beauty Express
Colds no More

Power drinks for radiant health ...

Whole, fresh natural foods are loaded with phytochemicals, powerful antioxidants and life-giving enzymes that re-activate the body's cells vital healing potential. Drinks made from nuts, seeds, vegetables and fruits are rich in nutrients that can easily be used by the human body. Containing no artificial substances, preservatives, fillers or binders, whole fresh organic foods can burn clean energy fuel within the body leaving no harmful toxins behind. When I make juices, shakes or smoothies I use only organic fruits and vegetables to ensure that I receive the full nutritional spectrum, without any nasty toxins, pesticides or heavy metal contaminants.

about nutty milks ...

I love the taste of nutty milks and my kids go crazy for these. Nutty milks can be made from any nut or seed. As a child I watched TV advertising campaigns proclaiming how milk gives you strong bones and teeth. This advertising was probably true back in the seventies when milk was less tampered with. However, most of the milk available today is highly pasteurized and homogenized. Pasteurization is the process of heating milk at high temperatures to kill germs. Unfortunately it kills not only the germs, but also beneficial bacteria and nutrients like iodine found in milk. The calcium found in this type of milk is difficult to absorb, so instead of giving you strong bones and teeth as the add suggests, it can actually lead to middle ear infections, tonsillitis, asthma, bone spurs and weak teeth. I am not against cow's milk, I simply think that once it is exposed to high temperatures it is not a living food anymore. If you wish to drink cow's milk, I would suggest 'raw milk' which is labeled 'bath milk - not fit for human consumption'. I know it is cheeky to say, but I believe authorities should swap the labels and put the 'not fit for human consumption' on the right milk.

For a healthier option, why not try making your own nut and seed milks. They are high in minerals like magnesium, phosphorous and calcium and contain protein to boost immunity, energy and healing. I often add celtic salt to my nutty milks to boost their mineral content even more. Nut milks can be used on cereals, in smoothies or in any dish to give a creamier texture. It is important to use a good industrial blender when making nut milks otherwise you won't break down the nuts well. I also put my nutty milks through a fine sieve or cheesecloth to keep the milk creamy and grain free. In most of my nutty milks I use medjool dates to sweeten, however, you can always use prunes, figs, stevia, xylitol, yacon syrup or another natural sweetener. To change the flavor of your nut milk, simply change the nuts or seeds used.

healing properties of nuts ...

Almonds contain huge amounts of protein, fibre, magnesium, manganese, copper, riboflavin, folic acid and Vitamin E. They are high in healthy monounsaturated fats to lower cholesterol and rich in potassium to lower blood pressure. An average serve of almond milk can supply 30% of our daily calcium needs and 25% of our Vitamin D needs to strengthen bones. The huge amount of Vitamin E found in this little nut protects against heart disease and cancer and the Vitamin A guards against infections and eye problems. The healthy fats found in almonds are famous for beautifying the skin and enhancing weight loss.

Brazil nuts are rich in monounsaturated fats to lower the 'bad' cholesterol and raise the 'good' cholesterol. They contain one of the highest sources of selenium to protect against cancer. They are rich in Vitamin E to protect the heart and contain good amounts of Vitamin B1, B2, B3, B5, B6 and folate to calm the nerves, enhance digestion and boost energy. Brazils are high in copper, magnesium, manganese, calcium, iron and zinc and they contain all amino acids, making them ideal for vegetarians.

Cashews are rich in iron, selenium, phosphorous, zinc, protein, antioxidants and healthy oils. They guard against several forms of cancer, including colon cancer. The cashew is definitely a 'heart smart' nut. It is low in fat, high in healthy oleic acid fats and rich in magnesium to lower cholesterol and blood pressure, while protecting against heart disease. This nut's rich copper content can improve the elasticity of collagen and elastin, improving joint, cartilage and skin health. This little nut can also prevent gallstones.

Walnuts, just a quarter of a cup, can supply 95% of your daily needs of omega 3 fatty acids. These fats lower 'bad cholesterol' and raise 'good cholesterol', reducing your risk of strokes and heart attacks. These fats also protect against breast, colon and prostate cancer. Walnuts contain melatonin, ellagic acid, Vitamin E and carotenoids to slow down ageing, inflammation and neurological diseases. Walnuts have the highest antioxidant content of any nut – in fact only six walnuts per day can scavenge a vast array of disease causing free radicals. On top of this they are a brilliant source of B vitamins, copper, calcium and other minerals.

Hazelnuts are full of healthy monounsaturated fats like oleic acid. These fats lower 'bad' cholesterol and raise 'good' cholesterol, reducing the risk of strokes and heart attacks. Hazelnuts contain the powerful proanthocyanins - quercetin and kaempferol. These flavonoids, which are also found in green tea, help to protect against allergies, neurological problems and cancer. One third of a cup of hazelnuts can supply up to one third of the body's iron needs, as well as magnesium, potassium, folate, B1, B2, B6 and Vitamin E. Hazelnuts supply beta-sitosterol to guard against prostate enlargement and cancer. Hazelnut milk with its rich protein, iron and Vitamin E content is a fantastic remedy for anemia and reproductive problems. The natural oils found in this magical nut beautify and tone the skin while improving skin elasticity and texture.

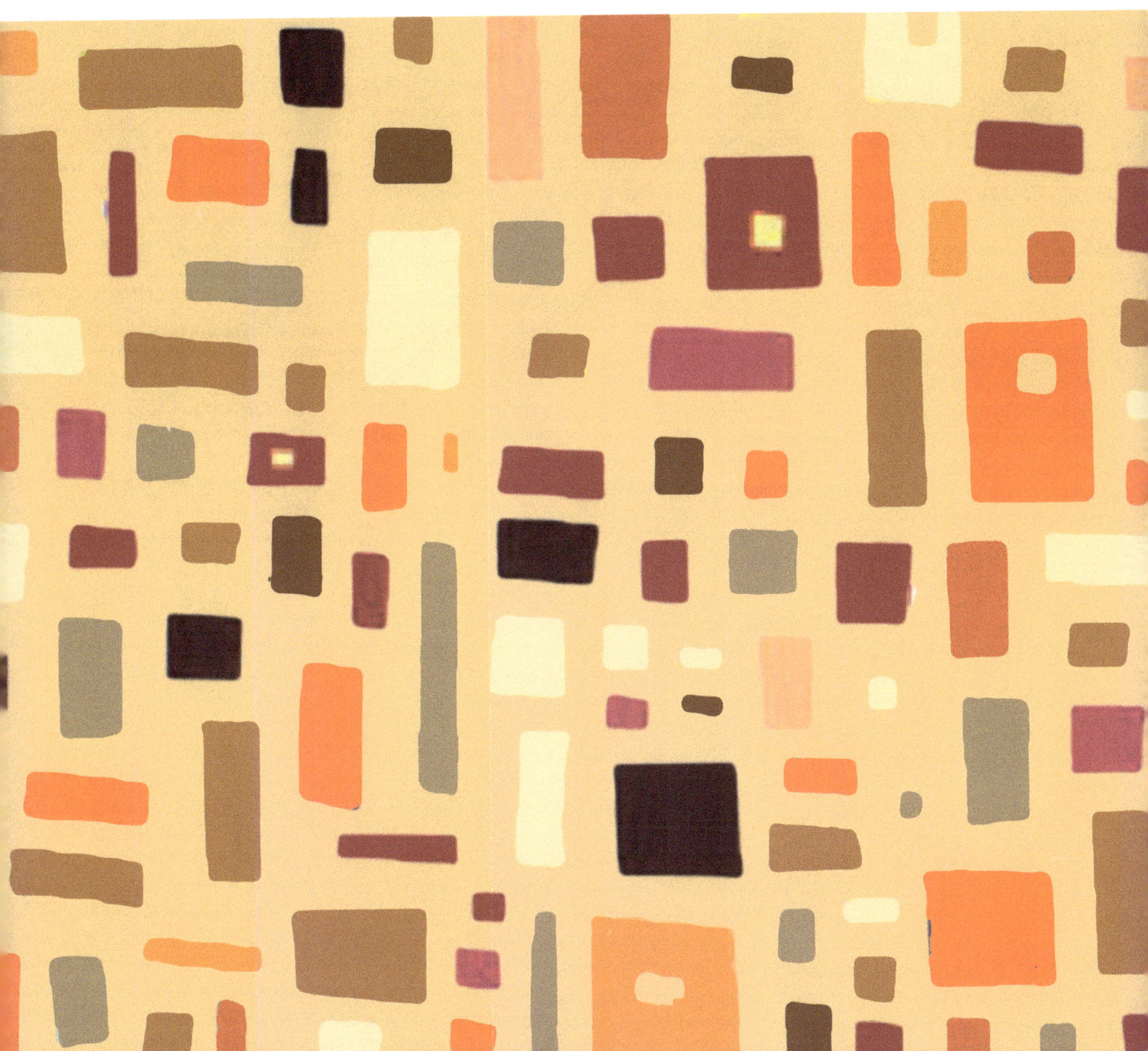

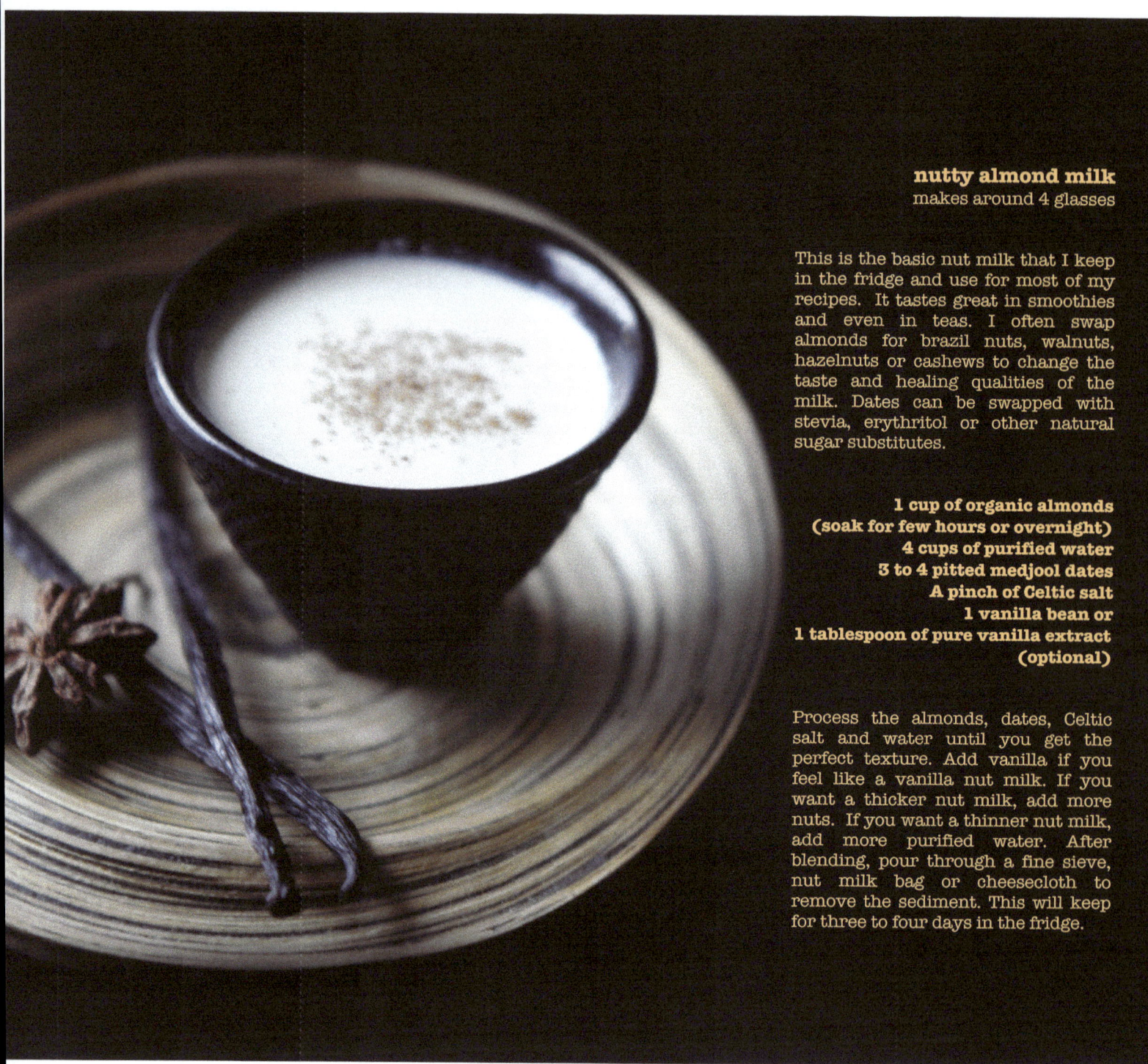

nutty almond milk
makes around 4 glasses

This is the basic nut milk that I keep in the fridge and use for most of my recipes. It tastes great in smoothies and even in teas. I often swap almonds for brazil nuts, walnuts, hazelnuts or cashews to change the taste and healing qualities of the milk. Dates can be swapped with stevia, erythritol or other natural sugar substitutes.

1 cup of organic almonds
(soak for few hours or overnight)
4 cups of purified water
3 to 4 pitted medjool dates
A pinch of Celtic salt
1 vanilla bean or
1 tablespoon of pure vanilla extract
(optional)

Process the almonds, dates, Celtic salt and water until you get the perfect texture. Add vanilla if you feel like a vanilla nut milk. If you want a thicker nut milk, add more nuts. If you want a thinner nut milk, add more purified water. After blending, pour through a fine sieve, nut milk bag or cheesecloth to remove the sediment. This will keep for three to four days in the fridge.

vanilla hazelnut swirl ...
makes 3 to 4 glasses

1 cup of hazelnuts (soak for a few hours or overnight to soften)
3 to 4 pitted, medjool dates
1 vanilla bean (open seeds and use) or 1 tablespoon of pure vanilla extract
1 ripe banana
A pinch of Celtic salt
3 to 4 cups of purified water
1 to 2 tablespoons of tahini (optional)

Put the hazelnuts, banana, dates, vanilla bean, salt and water into a food processor or blender and mix until creamy. Pour through a sieve to remove the grainy texture. To power up this nut milk with more B vitamins and minerals, blend with one tablespoon of nutritional yeast and tahini.

berry mocha ...
makes 3 glasses

3 cups of hazelnut, cashew or almond milk (recipe above)
1 cup of strawberries or freshly pitted cherries
2 to 3 pitted, medjool dates
1 vanilla bean or 1 tablespoon of pure vanilla extract
2 tablespoons of organic cacao powder (or a mix of cocoa and cacao)
1 tablespoon of coconut oil
ice

Blend nut milk with strawberries or cherries, dates, vanilla, cacao or cocoa, oil and water until smooth. I love this blended with ice.

miracle fruit ...

Cherries have one of the highest ORAC values (over 12000) of any fruit. They contain 17 antioxidants that help to fight disease and ageing. The anthocyanins found in cherries are capable of reducing high amounts of inflammation linked to arthritis, gout and other inflammatory conditions. Cherries also contain melatonin, a neurotransmitter which can help the body find the perfect sleep-wake cycle, great news for anyone with insomnia or sleeping problems. Cherries are one of the best anti-cancer fruits found on the planet – so don't forget to add cherries to your shopping list.

hazelnut cinnamon
makes 2 to 3 glasses

2 cups of hazelnut milk
1 teaspoon of raw activated honey or yacon syrup
1 teaspoon of pure cinnamon or twigs

Blend hazelnut milk with raw honey or yacon syrup and cinnamon. I love this drink warmed up in winter. Heat up gently on a stove (keep below 116 F or 46 C) or in a dehydrator. For extra nutrition, add a little celtic salt and tahini.

chocaholic
makes 3 glasses

3 cups of nutty almond milk
1 tablespoon of cacao powder
1 tablespoon of cocoa powder
a pinch of Celtic salt
2 to 3 pitted medjool dates
¼ teaspoon of cinnamon powder (optional)

Blend the nutty almond milk with dates, cocoa and/or cacao, Celtic salt and cinnamon until smooth. To get a smooth nut milk, pour through a sieve or nut milk bag. For milk chocolate lovers, use only cocoa powder and for dark chocolate lovers use only cacao powder. For an even healthier choc milk, mix half mesquite powder with half cacao powder.

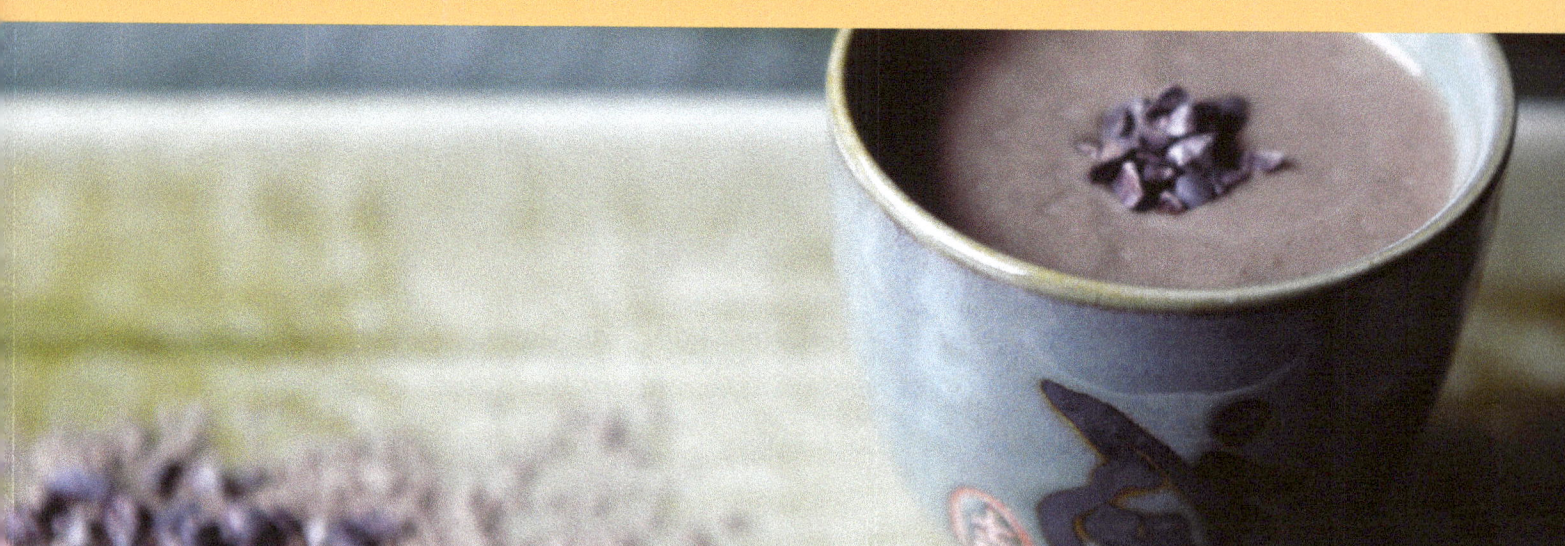

These are my super fruit smoothies, full of delicious fruit combinations. I always choose fruit with the highest antioxidant and phytonutrient content to ensure that my smoothie combinations are not only delicious, but brimming with nutrition. If you want icier summer creations, freeze fruit like mangoes, bananas and berries. Fruits are natural body cleansers that provide quick sources of energy and plenty of healing antioxidants.

super fruit smoothies ...

mango tango ...
makes 2 to 3 cups

4 tablespoons of almond or cashew yoghurt (or coconut yoghurt)
2 mangoes, cubed (great pre-frozen)
3 pitted medjool dates or 1 tsp of stevia or xylitol
1 vanilla bean or 1 tablespoon of pure vanilla extract
2 green apples
2 cups of purified water
lots of ice

If you don't have time to make nut yoghurt, use sugar free coconut yoghurt, or leave the yoghurt out and replace with more ice. Blend all of the ingredients in a processor. To change the flavour of this drink, simply change the fruit used. I often swap the mango for raspberries or pineapple and mint. This drink is so refreshing on a hot day – and brilliant for your digestion.

1 frozen banana
1 cup of fresh pineapple
1 cup of young coconut water or fresh coconut meat
1 mango, cubed
2 cups of purified water
ice

dance in the tropics ...
makes around 3 cups

For a little taste of the tropics, you cannot go past this island vibe smoothie. Simply blend pineapple, mango, coconut meat or water with banana, water and ice. This drink is rich in minerals, flavonoids, enzymes and antioxidants to reduce inflammation, improve digestion and boost energy. If mango is out of season, simply leave out.

2 cups of chopped pineapple
½ cup of blueberries
½ cup of red grapes
1 green apple
handful of mint
one inch piece of ginger
1 lime (skin on)
2 to 3 cups of purified water

immune booster ...
makes 2 to 3 cups

Blend pineapple, blueberries, grapes, green apple, ginger, mint and lime with water and ice. This smoothie contains good amounts of Vitamin C, anthocyanins, ellagic acid, d-limonene, tannins and resveratrol to guard against cancer, viruses, infections and heart problems. It is brilliant for strengthening veins and capillaries and improving eyesight.

¼ watermelon, diced
1 lime (use a small amount of skin)
1 cup of strawberries
1 cup of purified water
ice

melon madness ...
makes 3 cups

Blend all of the ingredients together for a delicious energy-boosting smoothie. Watermelon is one of the best sources of Vitamin A, C and the powerful antioxidant, lycopene. Lycopene guards against sunburn and many different types of cancer including melanoma, prostate, lung, endometrial, colorectal and breast cancer.

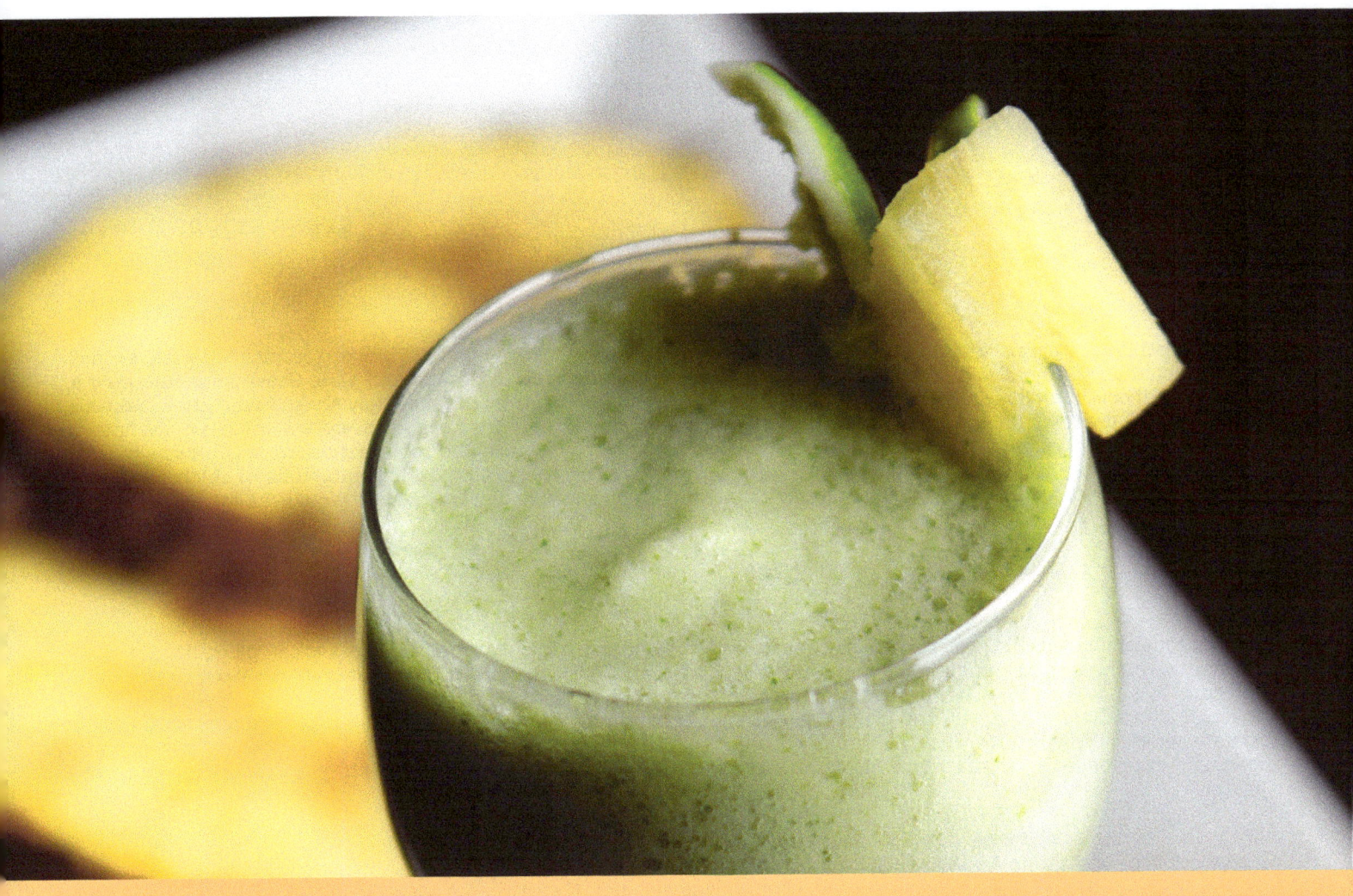

pine-lime punch
makes 3 cups

Process all ingredients together in a blender to make a delicious, summery fruit smoothie that is naturally alkalizing and full of healing antioxidants

- 3 cups of pineapple
- 1 lime (skin on)
- 1 green apple
- a handful of mint
- 1 to 2 cups of purified water

green smoothies ...

Green smoothies are green vegetables and fruits blended to make a nutritious drink. They are similar to juices, except they also contain the fibre and other healing nutrients from the food's stems, seeds and skin. Green smoothies are a superb way of obtaining huge amounts of nutrition and fibre, in one small glass. Because they are so filling, they make an ideal choice for breakfast. Many green smoothie recipes include lots of fruits, whereas my green smoothie recipes have a larger emphasis on green vegetables. Fruit contains large amounts of fructose and too much fructose can raise insulin levels leading to weight gain, diabetes and other problems. Green vegetables contain huge amounts of chlorophyll and healing nutrients to reduce ageing, enhance detoxification and prevent disease which is why I love to use them.

victorious vegetables ...

Spinach contains at least 12 well known anti-cancer and anti-inflammatory substances. It is a great 'blood builder' that boosts iron, calcium, potassium, magnesium, zinc, Vitamin C and carotenoid levels. These substances protect against eye problems, cataracts and macular degeneration. One cup of spinach can supply at least 20% of the body's fibre needs to prevent constipation, weight gain and blood sugar swings. Studies have shown its potential in guarding against skin and prostate cancer. Did you know that one cup of spinach also supplies over 337% of the RDA of Vitamin A - that is truly amazing - no wonder it boosts white bloods to fight disease. And to top this off, spinach is a brilliant anti-wrinkle vegetable.

Watercress is rich in sulfer based compounds called glucosilinates. These substances can block cancer formation. It is a fantastic source of Vitamin A to bolster immunity and protect the lungs against damage. This mustardy tasting vegetable is a great source of Vitamin B1, B2, B6, C, phosphorous and calcium. Watercress is a good source of iodine, so if you are suffering from a sluggish thyroid, don't forget to throw this zesty vegetable into your smoothie.

Kale is a superstar in the antioxidant and phytonutrient world. It contains more than 45 different anti-cancer flavonoids, including kaempferol and quercetin, Vitamin A and C, manganese, calcium, chlorophyll and indoles. Kale is the 'king' of cancer-preventing vegetables - it guards against breast, colon, bladder, gastric, ovarian and prostate cancer. One cup of kale supplies 36 calories and 0 grams of fat making it perfect for weight loss. The glucosinolates in kale stimulates liver detoxification. Kale provides a whopping dose of Vitamin K (over 1327% of the RDA) to strengthen bones and maintain brilliant health. No wonder kale is my favourite leafy green.

Broccoli is rich in d-glucaric acid, sulforaphane and indoles. Sulforaphane protects against the helicobacter pylori bacteria – a major cause of heartburn and gastric cancer. Indoles protect against many forms of cancer including lung, liver, colon, cervical, endometrial, prostate and breast cancers. D-glucaric acid is a powerful detoxifying substance that can remove dangerous hormones and substances that cause disease.

Cabbage is similar to kale and broccoli in its healing capacity. It can protect against lung, stomach, colon, prostate and breast cancer. It excretes harmful forms of estrogen and guards vigilantly against radiation toxicity. Cabbage juice is one of the best remedies for stomach ulcers.

Cucumbers are brilliant for hydration as they are almost 95% water. Their rich silica and sulphur content encourages hair growth, healthy joints and beautiful skin. They contain 3 powerful lignans which help to prevent prostate, breast, uterine and ovarian cancer. Cucumbers are the perfect remedy for hangovers and headaches because of their high vitamin and electrolyte levels. They are a brilliant weight loss vegetable.

Celery contains plenty of calcium, magnesium, potassium and pthalides to help lower high blood pressure and cholesterol. It is a great anti-inflammatory vegetable that eases gout, asthma and arthritis. Celery improves kidney function and prevents kidney stones, fluid retention and gallstones. It contains plenty of anti-cancer compounds to guard against stomach and colon cancer. For anyone suffering from constipation, high acidity, insomnia or sugar cravings, celery would be the perfect addition for you.

Lettuce - Iceberg lettuce isn't a brilliant source of nutrition, but most other darker coloured lettuces are. This is why it is great to eat mixed lettuces like endive, chicory, romaine lettuce and others. If the lettuce is dark, it will contain good amounts of Vitamin A, C, K and minerals. The darker lettuces are also quite high in iron and magnesium to nourish the nerves, muscles and blood. They also contain plenty of calcium to strengthen bones, potassium to lower blood pressure and sulphur, silica and phosphorous to promote creativity and improve the quality and beauty of the hair, skin and nails.

super green
makes 2 to 3 cups

This super green smoothie can be made without the banana if preferred. Add the banana if you want a slightly sweeter tasting green smoothie or otherwise add a pitted medjool date. This smoothie is alkalizing, detoxifying and full of energy - boosting and disease - preventing phytonutrients

½ avocado
1 banana (preferably frozen)
1 celery stalk with leaves
1 small organic lemon (skin on)
2 cups of mixed lettuce or spinach leaves
a handful of parsley
2 to 3 cups of purified water
ice (optional)

digestive-ease
makes 2 to 3 cups

1 cup of wheatgrass
1 cup of mixed lettuce
½ cup of paw paw (red or orange)
1 cup of sweet pineapple
a handful of mint
2 cups of purified water

If you cannot get fresh wheatgrass, use cabbage instead. Blend the ingredients in a food processor or blender. This smoothie is great for anyone with digestive problems, it contains chlorophyll to oxygenate the digestive tract, papain to digest proteins, and carbohydrates, fats, and mint to ease nausea and bloating

go for gold
makes 2 to 3 cups

3 large kale leaves
2 cups of baby spinach leaves
⅛ cup of fresh parsley
½ cucumber, skin on
1 mango (preferably frozen)
a handful of mint leaves
2 to 3 cups of purified water

Throw ingredients into a good processor and blend until smooth This is a superb blood purifying formula that is great for dull skin, fatigue, and fluid retention

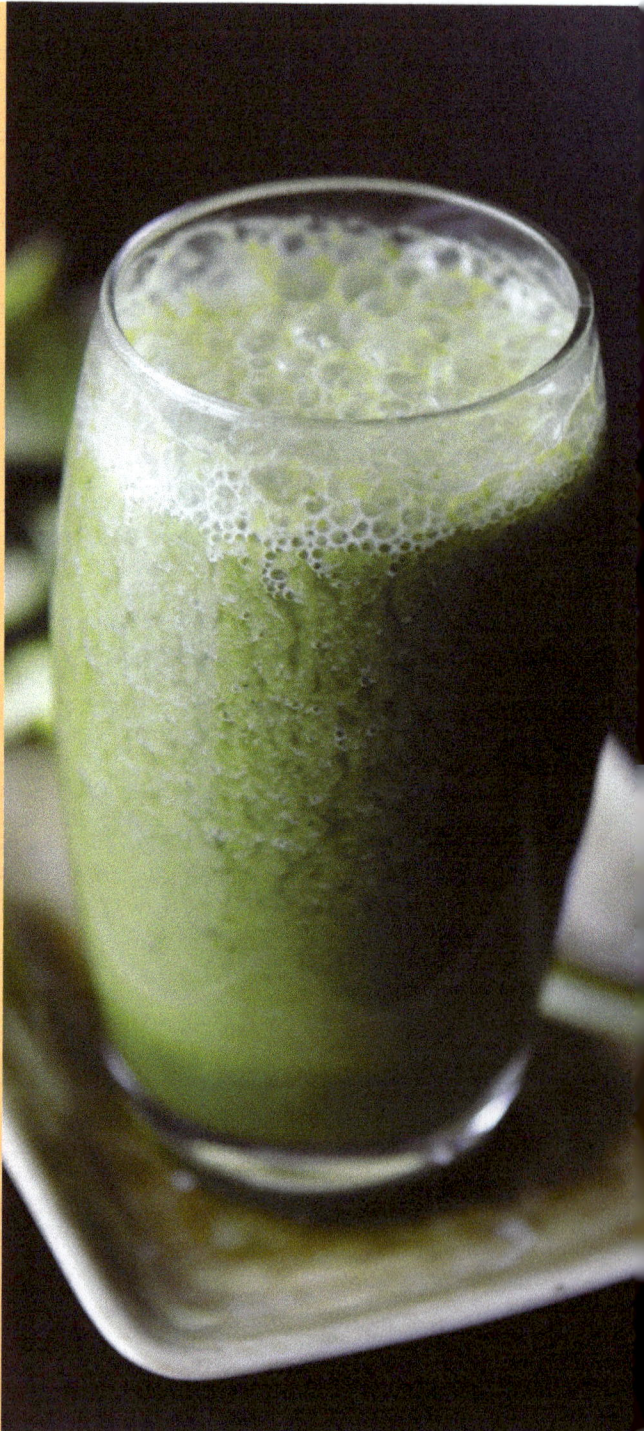

supermodel skin ...

4 to 5 leaves of romaine lettuce
1 cup of baby spinach leaves
1 cucumber (skin on)
1 cup of fresh pineapple
1 orange
½ red capsicum (optional)
2 to 3 cups of purified water

makes 2 cups

Process all of the ingredients until smooth. This drink contains huge amounts of silica, chlorophyll, enzymes and vitamins to boost collagen production protecting the skin against ageing and breakdown.

citrus peel - the ultimate healer... peels from lemons, limes and oranges contain an important anti-cancer ingredient called d-limonene. This substance is famous for helping to prevent breast, liver, colorectal and pancreatic cancer

for the love of green ...

2 cups of sweet, fresh pineapple
½ cup of blueberries
1 small lime (use some of the skin)
2 cups of baby spinach leaves
A handful of mint
2 cups of purified water
ice

makes 2 to 3 cups

Blend all ingredients in a processor or good blender. This smoothie tastes like a tropical mocktail. It will make your skin and eyes glow with vitality and is a perfect solution for boosting low iron levels.

no #1 green smoothie ...

1 mango (try using frozen mango pieces)
if not in season, replace with apple
1 frozen banana
3 to 5 kale leaves
1 cup of baby spinach leaves
A small bunch of parsley
2 cups of purified water

makes 2 to 3 cups

I call this my number 1 green smoothie as it is one of my favourite blends. Process all of the ingredients and drink straight away. I often add flaxseed meal and a super food green blend to this mix.

fantastic fruits ...

Papaya contains papain, an enzyme that improves digestion and guards against stomach and colorectal cancer. The huge amounts of folate found in this delicious fruit boosts red blood cell production giving good protection against cervical dysplasia and cancer. Chewing papaya seeds are one of the best remedies for killing worms.

Pineapple contains bromelain, a protein digeting enzyme that prevents bloating, gas and heartburn, as well as providing some amazing anti-inflammatory and anti-clotting actions. It can prevent strokes, relieve arthritis and heals sporting injuries and bursitis. It is a brilliant anti-ageing fruit rich in alpha-hydroxy acids (AHA's) to remove dead skin cells revealing a fresh, youthful skin.

Avocadoes were once called 'alligator pear' as they were found growing in the swamplands of South America. They are full of healthy monounsaturated fats that prevent obesity, cardiovascular disease and skin conditions like psoriasis and eczema. The green colour comes from its rich chlorophyll content which makes it a superb anti-cancer fruit. Avocadoes also contain lutein and Vitamin E to prevent wrinkles and improve the texture and quality of your skin and hair.

Grapes contain ellagic acid, a substance that can destroy cancer cells and protect against carcinogenic substances. Many red grapes are also rich sources of a powerful antioxidant resveratrol. Resveratrol protects the cells and heart against damage that causes cancer and cardiovascular disease.

Pomegranate contains an amazing array of antioxidants and cancer fighting nutrients including ellagic acid, flavonoids, tannins and Vitamin C. It props up immunity to fight several forms of cancer, including prostate cancer. This powerful fruit is a great heart protector.

Bananas rich potassium and magnesium levels help to protect against circulatory problems. They remove poisonous wastes from the kidneys, leaving a clean bloodstream. They contain pectin, a water soluble fibre that stops sugar cravings while removing toxins from the colon. They are brilliant for constipation, diarrhea, ulcers and fatigue. Bananas are a superb source of Vitamin A, C, E, B1, B2, B3, B5 and B6. No wonder apes go crazy for this little power fruit.

Lemons and **Limes** are a brilliant source of phosphorous. This mineral promotes creativity, improves memory and repairs the nervous system. Lemons also contain good amounts of sodium to eliminate wastes, cleanse the lymphatic system and liver and prevent hardened arteries. Lemons and limes are alkalizing fruits. If you need to reduce your acid levels, start adding some fresh lemon and lime juice to your water.

Apples are a rich source of the 'youth mineral' – potassium. Potassium softens hardened arteries, lowers blood pressure, boosts energy and prevents wrinkles. Apples also contain good amounts of pectin to remove wastes, prevent constipation and guard against stomach and colorectal cancer.

Mangoes contain lots of enzymes, bioflavonoids and Vitamin C to give protection against cancer. They contain ancardiol and anacadic, two powerful mood-uplifting substances and their rich Vitamin A levels help to guard against infections and eye problems.

Strawberries are full of Vitamin C, K, B2, B5, B6, folate, iodine, magnesium, omega 3 fats and plenty of antioxidant and anti-inflammatory substances like anthocyanins, ellagic acid, resveratrol, quercetin and kaempferol. No wonder strawberries are considered a superb anti-cancer and cardiovascular protecting super fruit. They powerfully fend off breast, cervical, colon and esophageal cancer.

Blueberries definitely rate high when it comes to antioxidant content. They contain huge amounts of anthocyanins, Vitamin E, A and B complex, selenium, zinc and iron. They can lower cholesterol, improve heart health, bolster immunity, prevent macular degeneration and even delay the ageing process. They promote circulation, repair capillaries and reduce inflammation. And to top this off, new studies have proven that blueberries can reduce tummy fat while controlling insulin resistance linked to diabetes and weight gain. They are definitely one of my favourite anti-ageing fruits. They contain pterostilbene, ellagic acid, luteolin, Vitamin C and other substances to guard against colon, liver, skin and ovarian cancer. No wonder I add blueberries to so many of my living food creations.

Pears are coined 'nature's perfect laxative'. They contain pectin to prevent constipation while dropping cholesterol. They also contain plenty of Vitamin A, B1, B2, B3, C and folate to prevent high blood pressure, infections and anemia.

bathroom bliss ...
makes 2 to 3 cups

1 cup of red or purple grapes
1 orange (use a little skin)
1 pear
2 cups of baby spinach, lettuce or cabbage
1 lebanese cucumber or zucchini (skin on)
1 tablespoon of flaxseed meal
2 prunes
3 cups of purified water
ice

Blend all of the ingredients in a food processor. If you are feeling blocked up – this smoothie is pure bathroom heaven.

These shakes are so healthy you will be running laps around the block! They contain plenty of 'power foods' to heal the body and power up your immune system to its greatest fighting potential. Even though they seem 'naughty', they are actually packed with a huge number of cancer-fighting antioxidants, minerals and vitamins to restore lost energy levels. You can use any nut milk as the base of your power shake or even organic soy milk, raw milk, rice milk or juice.

'SHAKE IT UP' power shakes ...

goji heaven
makes 3 glasses

1 cup of nut milk
(or swap for your own milk)
2 to 3 cups of purified water
1 tablespoon of pure cacao powder
1 tablespoon of mesquite powder
3 pitted medjool dates or
1 teaspoon of xylitol or yacon syrup
¼ cup of goji berries
1 tablespoon of freeze dried acai powder
1 tablespoon of unbleached lecithin granules
1 tablespoon of flaxseed meal
1 tablespoon of pure vanilla extract
or 1 vanilla pod (de-seeded)

Blend the nut milk, acai, vanilla, cacao, mesquite, natural sweetener, goji berries, flaxseed meal, lecithin and purified water and ice until smooth. Acai and goji are potent super foods famous for boosting energy, vitality, and longevity.

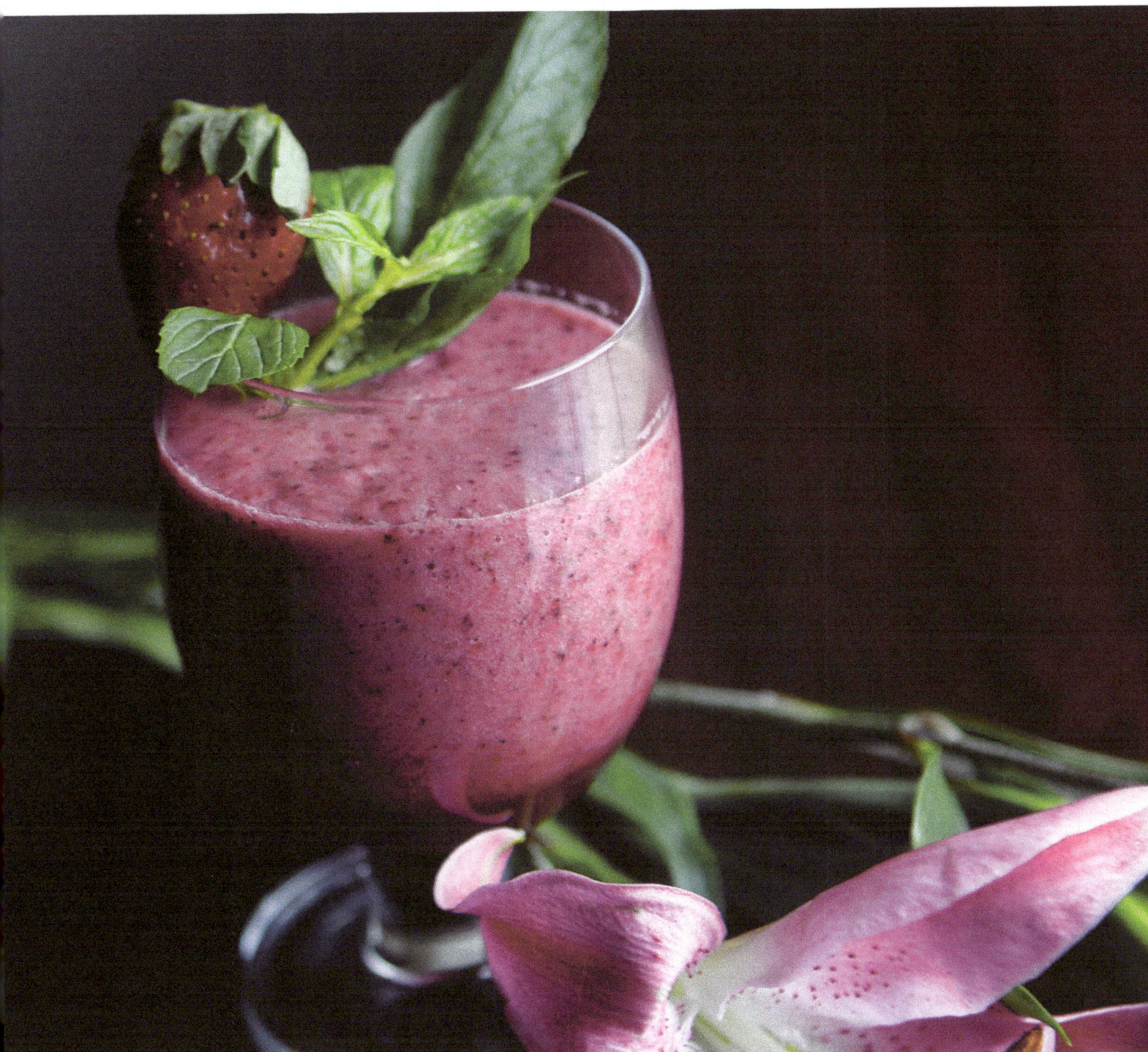

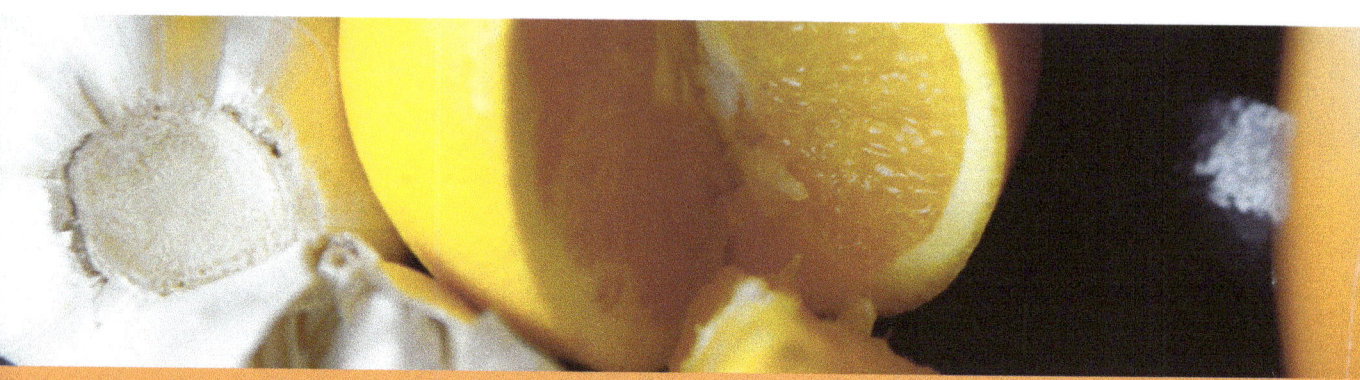

This is a my perfect 'anti-cancer' shake as it floods the body with cancer-fighting antioxidants to boost immunity, energy and metabolism. Blueberries contain pterostilbene to protect against colorectal cancer and anthocyanins to stop the onset, promotion and spread of cancer. Flaxseeds are brimming with omega 3 fatty acids and lignans to guard against breast, colon, prostate and ovarian cancer. Wheatgerm is full of Vitamin E to thin the blood, improve circulation and beautify the skin. Hemp seed protein is over 50% protein and contains every amino acid to repair, heal cells, DNA and tissues. Wow – no wonder I named this the 'cancer kicking power shake'.

cancer-kicking power shake
makes 2 to 3 glasses

1 teaspoon of pure colostrum powder
1 tablespoon of ground flaxseeds or pre-soaked flaxseeds
1 teaspoon of torula or brewer's yeast
1 teaspoon of lecithin granules
1 teaspoon of bee pollen granules
2 tablespoons of hemp seed oil
2 tablespoons of raw hemp seed protein powder
1 tablespoon of organic spirulina and wheatgrass powder
2 to 3 pitted medjool dates or 1 tsp of yacon syrup/xylitol or stevia
¼ cup of blueberries or raspberries or banana
1 cup of nut milk
2 cups of purified water

Blend all of the ingredients in a blender with ice
The world's strongest multi-vitamin could not even match the nutritional spectrum found in this power shake

superfood additions ...

Acai contains twice the antioxidant potential of blueberries, ten times the antioxidant level of grapes and ten to thirty times more anthocyanins than red wine – wow, no wonder it is nicknamed 'god's superfood'. The ORAC value for 100 grams of organic, freeze dried acai is over 70 000. That's amazing, especially when you consider that the average person consumes less than 1000 values of ORAC per day.

Barley Grass is taken from the barley before the grain has developed. It contains good amounts of chlorophyll, to boost oxygen levels, encourage detoxification and eliminate bad breath. It is a good source of vitamins, minerals, amino acids, beta-carotene and S.O.D (superoxide dismutase). SOD is a powerful substance that can help to detoxify harmful substances that cause cancer and ageing. Barley grass helps to prevent diabetes, arthritis and fatigue.

Colostrum is the first food derived from the 'let down' of a mother's milk. Supplemental colostrum is obtained from grass fed cows. It is a unique combination of immunoglobulins, antibodies, and immune enhancers designed to protect a baby against viruses, bacteria and allergens. Together with lactobacillus acidophilus colostrum can kick start the immune system to fight disease. It contains lactoferrin, a powerful immune stimulant that guards against food allergies and many different types of cancer, including lymphoma, leukemia and colon cancer.

Hemp seeds are one of nature's most perfect foods. The protein taken from these magical seeds contain all essential and non-essential amino acids, making it a superb source of nutrition to help boost immunity and energy. Hemp contains a perfect balance of omega 3 and 6 fatty acids, as well as plenty of phytonutrients to protect the cells, blood and organs against damage. Definitely one of my favourite super foods for restoring lost energy!

Lecithin is a combination of phospholipids and fatty acids that are normally taken from soybeans. It is brilliant for memory, fat and cholesterol reduction, liver function and nerve health. Lecithin makes phosphatidyl choline and serine, substances that can be beneficial for Epilepsy, Parkinson's and other neurological problems. A good source of lecithin is found in egg yolk.

Maca is a root vegetable grown 4000 metres above sea level in the Andes mountains. The Inca Indians have used this for close to two thousand years for its restorative and balancing powers on the endocrine system. It contains good amounts of Vitamin B1, B2, B12, C, E, zinc, magnesium, iron, calcium and protein. It can balance the pituitary, adrenals and ovaries/testicles to help with fertility, menopause, virility and hormone balance.

Royal Jelly is the nectar secreted from the glands of nurse bees. It is used to feed their 'queen' – hence the name, 'Royal Jelly'. Workers bees live for 4 to 6 weeks, whereas the queen can live for 5 to 8 years and lay up to 3000 eggs per day. The queens nutritious nectar, royal jelly, is thought to be responsible for her amazing virility and long life span. The nectar contains a gelatin that helps to make collagen. This keeps the skin looking radiant, youthful and wrinkle free. It is a rich source of lipids, protein, Vitamin A, C, E and D, sterols, choline and B vitamins.

Spirulina is a blue-green algae that was harvested by the Aztecs as a nourishing food staple, centuries ago. It is a natural body rejuvenator and energy booster that easily balances blood sugar levels. It contains good amounts of essential fatty acids, Vitamin B12, iron, protein, carotenes, selenium, enzymes, RNA and DNA. It protects the liver against damage and is very effective in weight loss programs.

Wheatgerm is a brilliant source of protein, B1, B6, choline, inositol, calcium, copper, magnesium, zinc, potassium, Vitamin K and E and coenzyme Q10. It boosts energy, balances blood sugar, protects the heart and works well with muscular dystrophy.

Wheatgrass is a magical grass, nicknamed the 'elixir of life' or 'plasma of youth'. It is no wonder as wheatgrass contains over one hundred healing nutrients. Thirty mls of fresh wheatgrass juice is equal in nutritional value to over one kilogram of fresh vegetables. It is almost 70% chlorophyll and is brilliant for detoxification, liver and kidney health and cancer protection.

... and this is only a small list of my favourite super-foods.

chocolate rocket fuel
makes 2 to 3 glasses

2 cups of nut milk or purified water
2 tablespoons of raw cacao powder or nibs
1 tablespoon of raw carob or cocoa powder
1 tablespoon of mesquite powder
2 tablespoons of hemp seed protein
1 tablespoon of pure, freeze dried acai berry powder
1 tablespoon of maca powder
2 pitted medjool dates or 1 tablespoon of xylitol/erythritol or stevia
1 teaspoon of organic cinnamon powder or twigs

Put all ingredients in a blender and blend until smooth. A delicious, yummy chocolate drink that will have you jumping out of your skin with energy and vitality

juice remedies ...

It is easy to make yummy juices simply by using sweet fruits like oranges, pineapple, mint, apples and pears. The juices below may not be sweet, but they are definitely packed with huge amounts of nutrition to encourage detoxification and enhance healing. Juices do not contain fibre like green smoothies, making them more cleansing in nature.

heavy metal detox juice ...

4 medium carrots
2 green apples
3 celery stalks
¼ head of cabbage
3 broccoli florets
a handful of coriander

Juice the carrots, celery, apples, coriander, cabbage and broccoli. Pour into a glass and serve. This is an amazing juice for detoxifying radioactive isotopes and heavy metals like mercury, arsenic, lead, aluminium and copper from the body. To make this even more delicious, juice with fresh oranges.

super 9 ..

2 kale leaves
1 celery stalk, use a few tops
1 carrot
1 tomato
¼ cup of baby spinach leaves
⅛ red capsicum
3 broccoli florets
1 small lemon
a handful of parsley

Juice all of the ingredients and chill for five minutes in the fridge. Mix well before drinking. This juice is full of healing phytonutrients and antioxidants like lycopene, quercetin, chlorophyll, Vitamin A, C and iron.

resveratrol treat

3 green apples
2 cups of red or purple grapes
½ cup of blueberries
1 chunk of ginger
1 lemon
2 tablespoons of flaxseeds (pre-soaked) or flaxseed meal

Juice the apples, grapes, ginger and lemon. Put the liquid into a blender with blueberries, flaxseed meal, ice and water. This drink is full of phytonutrients like Vitamin C, pectin and resveratrol. Resveratrol is a powerful antioxidant that guards against cardiovascular disease and prostate, breast, colon, pancreatic and thyroid cancers.

anti-cancer vitamin pill

3 medium carrots
2 small radish
½ beetroot
1 lemon (use a little skin)
a small chunk of fresh turmeric
3 kale leaves, silverbeet or spinach leaves
a handful of parsley

Juice all of the ingredients – add a little green apple if the taste is too overpowering. This juice contains curcumin, Vitamin A, C, E. d-limonene and other powerful ingredients to ward off infections, cancer and other diseases. This is a detoxifying, alkalizing and immune boosting super juice.

beauty express

2 cucumbers, skin on
½ cup of parsley
3 carrots
1 cup of romaine lettuce

Juice all of the ingredients for a pure skin smoothing and anti-wrinkle treat. Romaine lettuce is rich in chlorophyll, sulfur, chlorine, silica and B vitamins to improve hair growth and skin health. Cucumbers are full of silica to improve the texture, quality and elasticity of the skin.

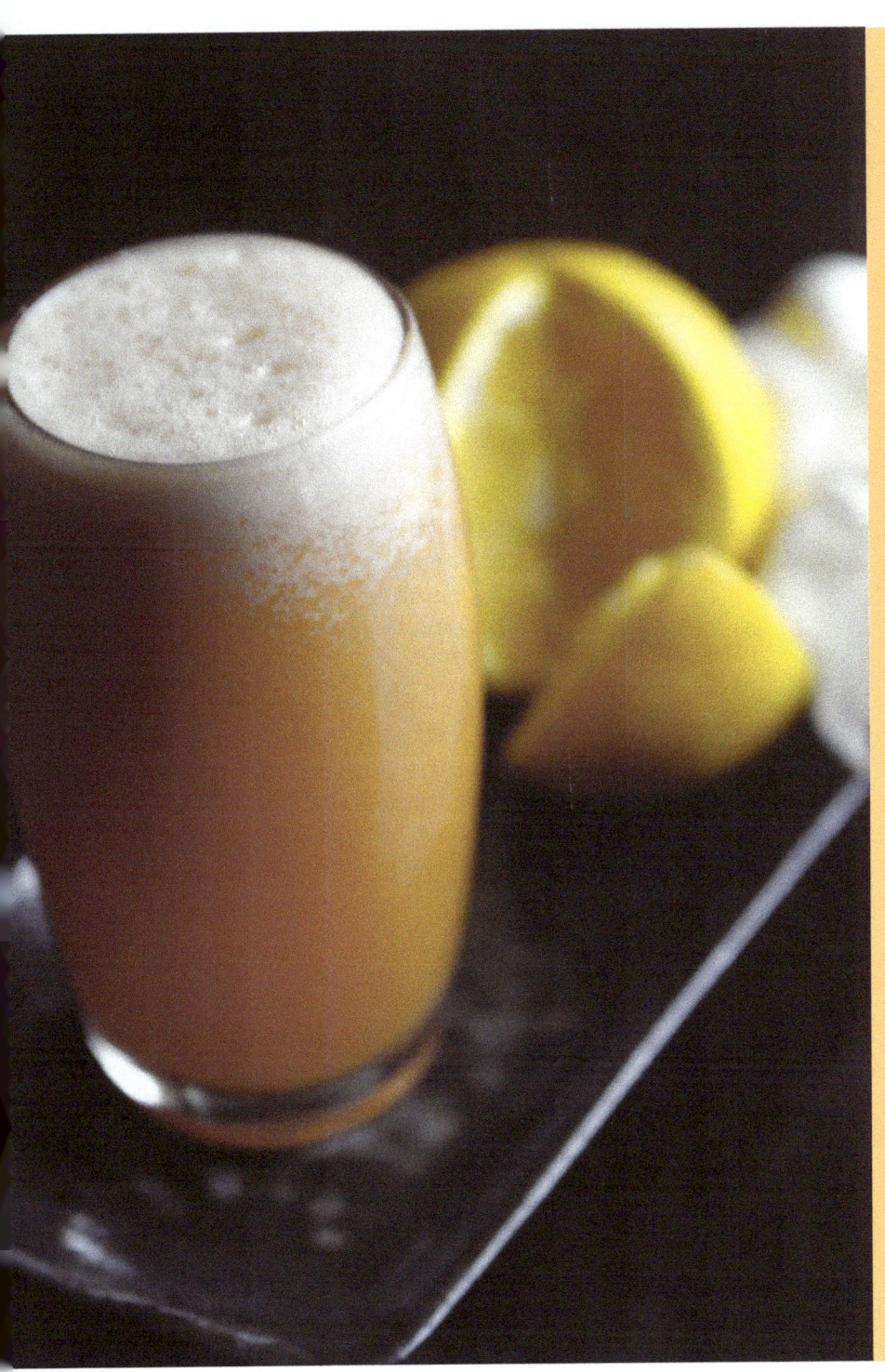

colds no more...

**3 medium carrots
1 lemon (use some skin)
2 cloves of garlic
a small chunk of ginger
2 oranges**

Juice all of the ingredients and drink immediately. If you are worried about the garlic on your breath, chew a little parsley or dill to freshen the breath. This juice contains Vitamin A, C and sulpher compounds to ward off colds, flu's and viruses.

Super Yummy Cereals
Banana Buckwheat Porridge
Goji Buckwheat Crunch
Mocha Almond Crunch
Tropical Buckwheat Crispies
Banana Chia Pudding
Blueberry Quinoa Delight
Energy Flax Muesli

Brekkie Whips and Yoghurts
Creamy Almond Yoghurt
Banana and Coconut Whip
Lemon and Vanilla Mousse
Green Apple, Honey and Mint Whip

Breakfast Scrambles
Healthy Scrambled "Not Eggs"
Oriental Scrambled "Not Eggs"
Mediterranean Scrambled "Not Eggs"
Mexican Scrambled "Not Eggs"

Breakfast Ideas ...

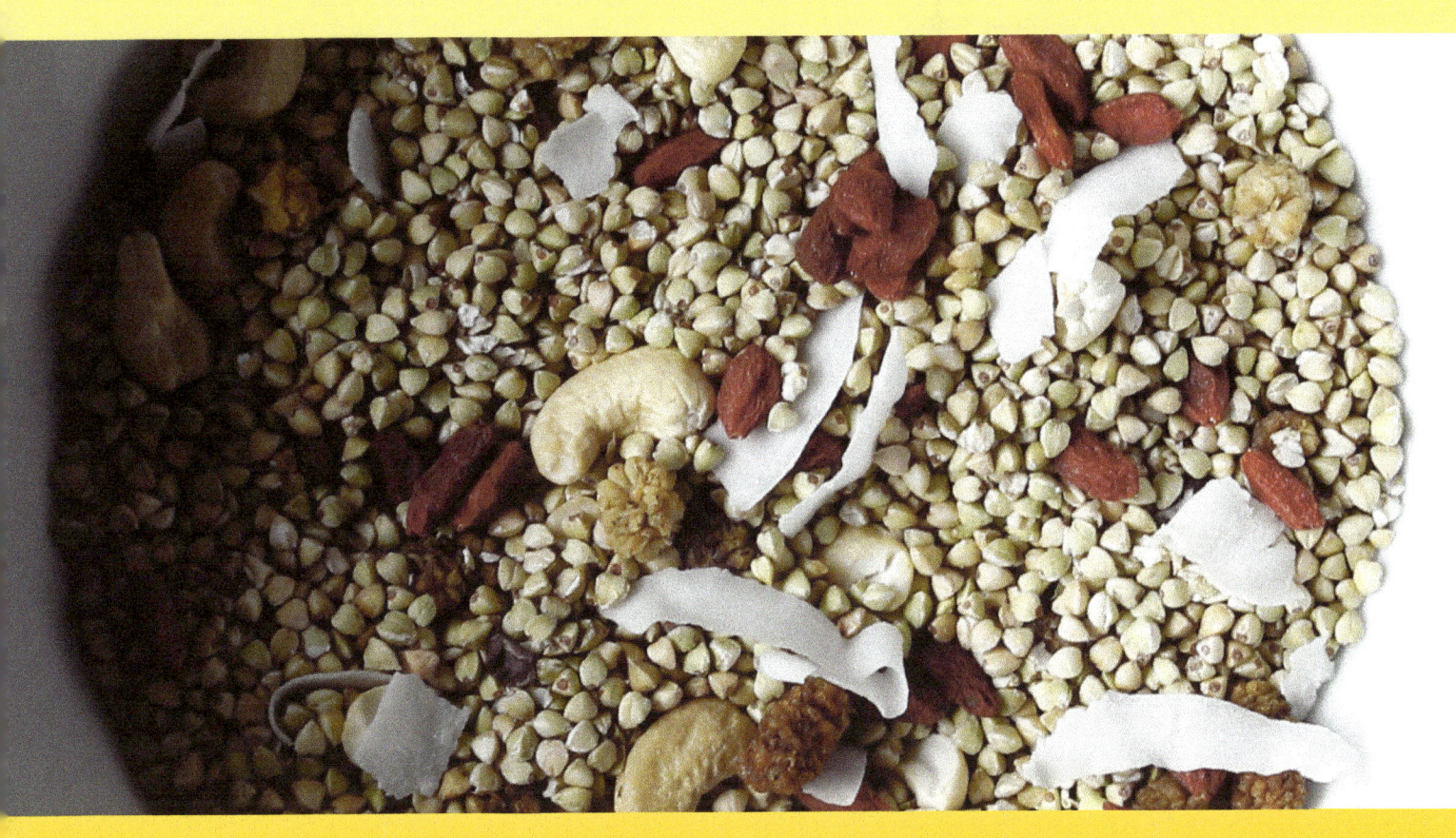

As a little girl I grew up in a traditional Australian household where the normal breakfast choices were weet-bix and corn flakes, omelettes, scrambled eggs, bacon and grilled cheese on toast. Sometimes if we felt a little exotic we would add avocado and fresh lemon juice to the toast. As my mum discovered the wonders of living foods our traditional 'aussie' breakfast definitely took on more exotic and creative flavours. When I was old enough to travel to foreign lands I then began to discover the wonder of eating fried rice, hot soups and steamed fish in the morning – food I would have previously thought of as only 'lunch' or 'dinner' meals.

I now love the concept of choosing foods based on nutrition, rather than based on traditional conditioning of 'set meal times'. Have you ever thought of having a yummy salad with creamy avocado, sprouts, activated nuts and lemon juice for breakfast? What about a breakfast 'no egg scramble'? This is just as yummy as scrambled eggs, except the eggs are replaced with highly nutritious nuts, seeds, herbs and spices. Another lighter option which I love is a green smoothie – a nutritious liquid blend of green vegetables and fruits. On the days I consult I often whip up a green smoothie made from baby spinach, kale, parsley, banana, flaxseed meal, blueberries and a super nutritious green food blend. It's a lighter option that gives me loads of energy for the day. Cereals are another good choice, especially if you get creative and make your own. I love using buckwheat, amaranth or quinoa as the base of cereals. I always soak my grains and sometimes dehydrate these to give them a lighter, crunchier texture. Breakfast doesn't have to be boring – it can be one of your yummiest and most creative meals of the day if you learn to experiment with the exotic flavours of raw foods.

breakfast toasties ..
Groats are from whole grains like barley, buckwheat and oats. They contain the cereal portion, the fibre and the endosperm, which is normally removed during processing. They are very hard so they need to be soaked to be eaten. They make a yummy, nutritious and crunchy base in cereal mixes. You can use any grain to make these toasties, but I would probably stick to buckwheat, brown rice, oats or barley to get a nice crunchy texture.

buckwheat crispies ...
500 grams of Buckwheat groats (or another grain)
Put buckwheat groats into a bowl and cover with water. Let this soak overnight and rinse every six to eight hours as the water can turn very slimy. From here you can either sprout the buckwheat or turn them into buckwheat crispies. To make crispies, spread the buckwheat onto mesh screens and dehydrate at 115 F or 42 C for six to 10 hours. If you don't have a dehydrator, toast in the oven at 250 C until crunchy. My daughter loves to eat these as a snack.

hot kitchen tip ...
I soak all of my nuts and seeds for five to eight hours in filtered water. I then rinse them well with filtered water. If you plan to add these to dry cereals, then dry off the nuts. If you decide to use these in wet cereals there is no need to dry them at all.

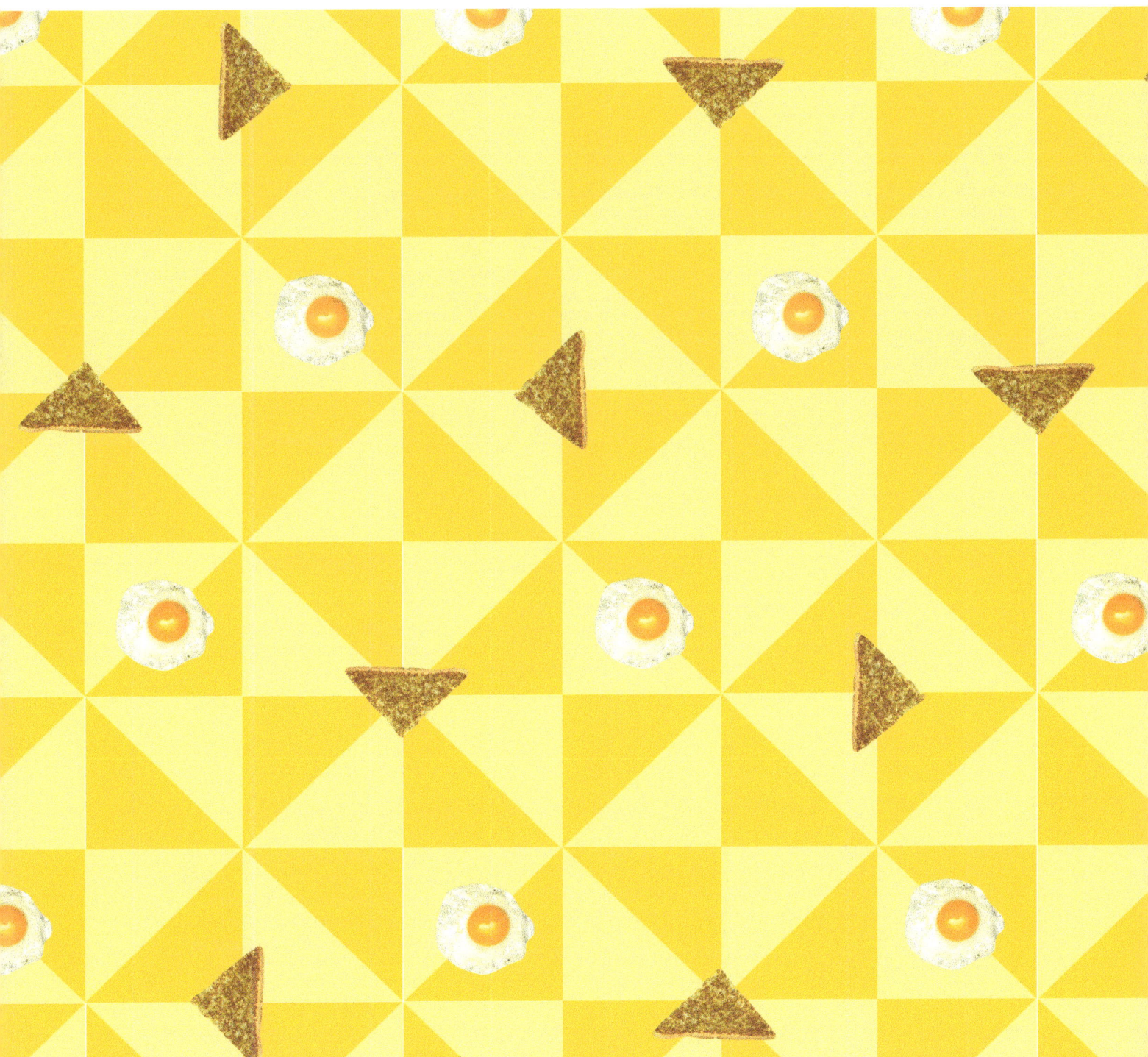

These super nutritious cereals are one of the few recipes within this book that take more than ten minutes to make. This is because I use the rawest and healthiest form of a whole grain called a 'groat'. Because groats are very hard they need to be softened by soaking. When they are soft, they can either be sprouted to increase their healing impact or dehydrated to add a crunchy texture to cereals. Dehydrated grains will keep for a long time in jars, so you can store and add to cereals as needed.

I also sweeten many of my cereal dishes with dates. Even though dates are higher in natural sugars, they contain plenty of healing nutrients and antioxidants to benefit health. An even healthier option is a medjool date. They are highly nutritious and large, so you only need two to three of these to add a lovely sweet flavour to a dish. If you are on a completely sugar free diet, swap dates for pure forms of stevia, xylitol or erythritol.

super yummy cereals ...

banana buckwheat porridge
makes 1 to 2 bowls

Place buckwheat crispies in a blender with nut milk or water, dates, sunflower seeds, cinnamon and banana to make a creamy buckwheat porridge. This is absolutely delicious in winter if you heat up in the dehydrator or on a stove keeping below 40 C

1 cup of buckwheat crispies
1 banana
¼ cup of nut milk or purified water
¼ cup of sunflower seeds
2 to 3 pitted medjool dates or ¼ cup of raisins
⅛ teaspoon of cinnamon

goji buckwheat crunch
makes 2 to 3 bowls

Stir together all of the ingredients and store in a glass jar in the fridge. When you are ready to eat place in a bowl and serve with your favourite milk. This cereal keeps the bowels regular and blood sugar levels balanced for exceptional weight loss and energy. If you don't have any buckwheat crispies on hand, leave out of the recipe and make a 'Goji Crunch' instead

2 cups of buckwheat crispies
¼ cup of flaxseed meal
¼ cup of lecithin granules
¼ cup of coconut chips or shredded coconut
¼ cup of organic goji berries
¼ cup of organic raisins
¼ cup of almonds (pre-soaked)

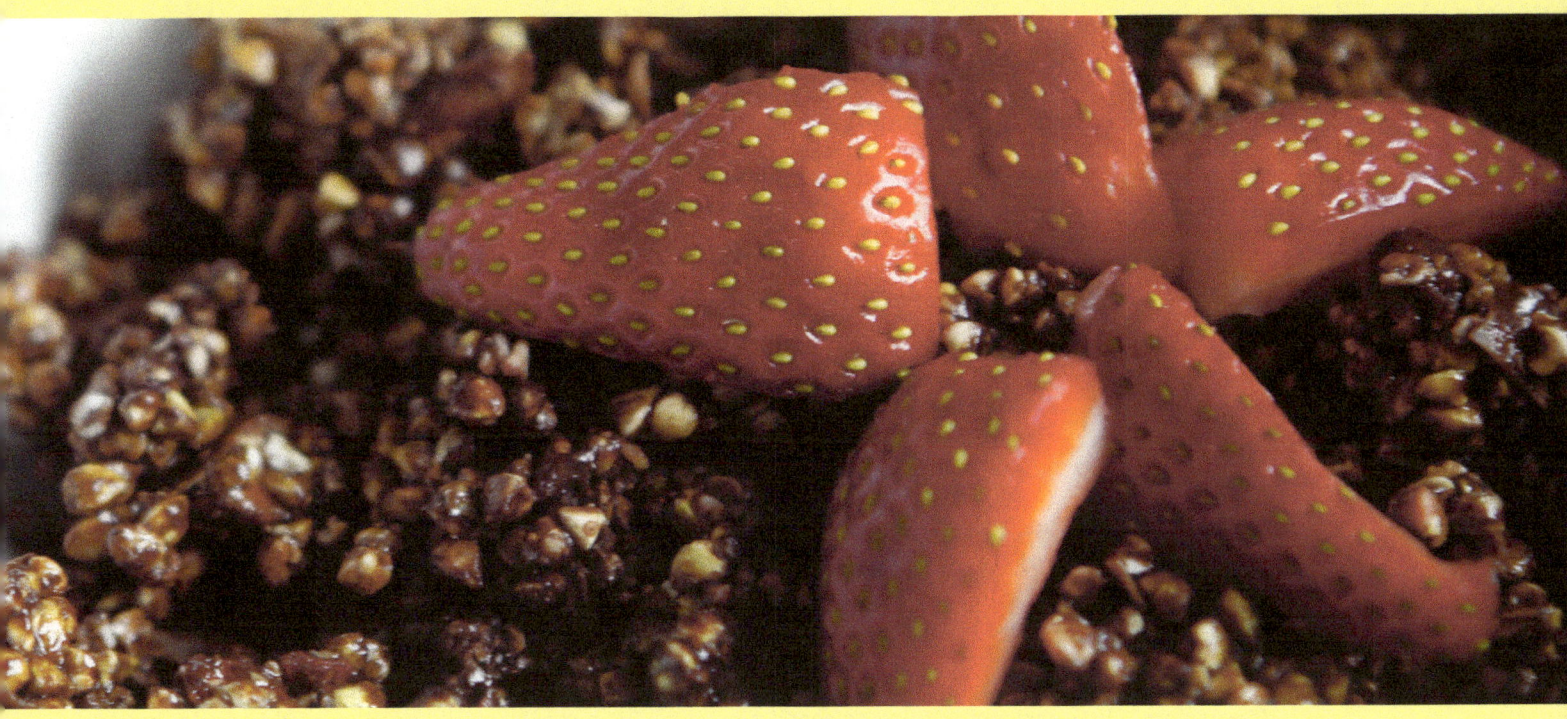

mocha almond crunch
makes 1 to 2 bowls

You can make this cereal in two different ways. Either mix all of the ingredients together in a bowl and serve with your favourite nut milk OR mix all of the ingredients together and spread onto teflex sheets. Dehydrate at 115 F or 46 C until crunchy, then turn over and cook on the other side. This is a decadent, yet nutritious treat that will keep for 3 days in the fridge. This can also be used as a healthy snack for kids.

- 2 cups of buckwheat crispies or sprouted, dehydrated quinoa
- 2 tablespoons of cacao powder
- 3 tablespoons of almond butter
- 1 tablespoon of mesquite
- 1 tablespoon of maca powder (optional)
- 2 tablespoons of agave or another natural sweetener
- ½ cup of goji berries
- ¼ cup of chopped almonds
- ¼ cup of coconut chips
- ½ teaspoon of cinnamon (optional)

Buckwheat crispies are easy to make and they store for weeks in the cupboard. If you don't have time to make these, you can always buy dehydrated buckwheat from your local health food store and replace in the recipes that call for 'buckwheat crispies'. Buckwheat is an alkaline grain that is very high in minerals like manganese, magnesium and copper and flavonoids like rutin. Rutin helps to guard against heart disease by preventing abnormal blood clotting, high cholesterol and high blood pressure. Buckwheat protects against breast cancer and other hormonally induced cancers. It prevents liver damage, boosts blood circulation, and aids diabetes.

tropical buckwheat crispies
makes 2 bowls

2 cups of buckwheat crispies
¼ cup of sunflower seeds
¼ cup of pecans or cashews
¼ cup of goji berries
¼ cup of dried white mulberries (optional - but yummy)
¼ cup of coconut chips (or shredded coconut)

Mix all of the ingredients together and put into two bowls. Serve with your favourite milk
If you want a little sweeter, add some cacao nibs and a little raw honey or yacon syrup and stir through

banana chia pudding
makes 1 to 2 bowls

¼ cup of cashews
2 tablespoons of chia seeds
3 pitted medjool dates
¼ teaspoon of cinnamon
2 tablespoons of lecithin granules
1 ripe banana
¾ cup of purified water

Blend all ingredients at a high speed until smooth and creamy. Add water to get the perfect texture
This tastes great with goji berries pulsed in at the end

blueberry quinoa delight ...
makes 1 to 2 bowls

- ½ cup of sprouted or dehydrated quinoa
- ½ cup of blueberries
- 1 small banana
- 1 tablespoon of flaxseed meal
- 1 tablespoon of shredded coconut
- ¼ cup of chopped walnuts
- 3 pitted medjool dates or 1 teaspoon of xylitol

Pulse sprouted quinoa with banana, flaxseed meal, shredded coconut, chopped walnuts and natural sweetener. Stir in fresh blueberries at the end. Serve with your favourite milk. If you don't have time to sprout quinoa, replace with puffed rice or amaranth flakes.

how to sprout and dehydrate quinoa ...

Rinse quinoa, cover with water and soak for thirty minutes. Drain, rinse, and return to wide mouthed jar. Cover jar with a cheesecloth and use a rubber band to hold in place. Put in a dark cool area. Rinse twice daily until the tails forms, which will take about 1 day. Wait until the tails are around ¼ inch long, rinse again and place in the fridge. To dehydrate, spread sprouted quinoa onto teflex sheets and heat at 115 F or 46 C for around five hours or until crunchy.

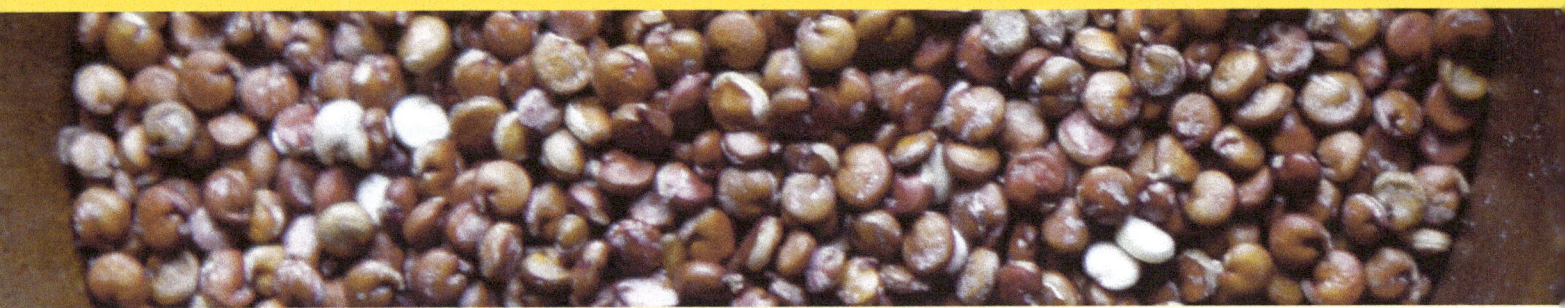

energy flax muesli

makes 2 to 3 bowls

2 cups of golden flaxseed meal
⅛ cup of lecithin granules
½ cup hulled hemp seeds
¼ cup of pumpkin seeds
¼ cup of chopped pecans
¼ cup of blackcurrants or goji berries
¼ cup of coconut chips
1 teaspoon of cinnamon
1 small banana, chopped
2 green apples, grated

Mix in a container flaxseed meal, lecithin granules, hemp seed, pecans, pumpkin seeds, cinnamon, coconut chips & currants or goji berries. To serve, place into a bowl and add some chopped banana and grated green apple. Use your favourite milk to flavour

brekkie whips and yoghurt ...

creamy almond yoghurt

makes 1 glass jar

1 cup of almonds (pre-soaked overnight or for a few hours)
1 cup of purified water
1 lemon, juiced

Blend almonds and lemon juice and gradually add enough water to get a yoghurt consistency. Pour into a muslin bag and squeeze out the liquid. Put this into a glass jar, cover with muslin or cheesecloth and let sit at room temperature for 8 hours then put in the fridge to set OR put a probiotic powder into the creamy mix and ferment the yoghurt in a dehydrator at 46 F for a short time, then place in the fridge. This will keep for 5 days in the fridge. I also love this yoghurt made from sprouted almonds, cinnamon and raw honey

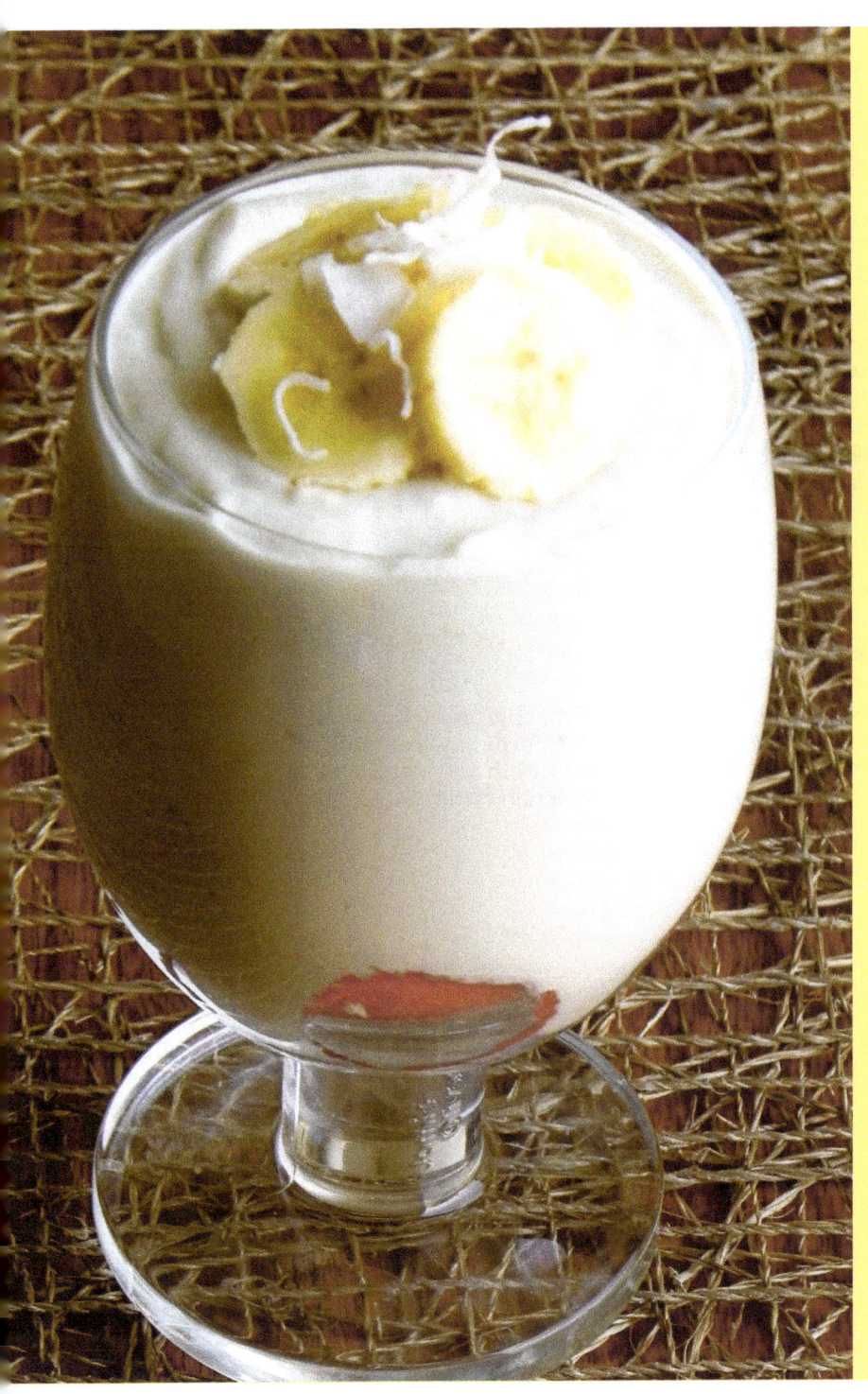

banana and coconut whip ...
makes 2 cups

**2 frozen bananas
½ cup of fresh coconut meat
(if you don't have fresh, use shredded)
2 tablespoons of lecithin granules
1 tablespoon of coconut oil
½ to 1 cup of purified water
1 cup of cashews**

Blend all of the ingredients adding more water if needed. Chill in the fridge or freezer until ready to eat. My daughter loves this as a snack after school. I often swap the coconut for mangoes in the summertime.

2 cups of almonds (soaked or sprouted) or 1 cup of almond meal
3 pitted medjool dates or 1 tbsp of yacon syrup or other
2 lemons, juiced
1 avocado
1 vanilla pod or 1 tablespoon of pure vanilla extract
2 tablespoons of lecithin granules
1 to 2 cups of purified water

lemon and vanilla mousse ...
makes 2 to 3 cups

Blend the almond meal, lemon juice, avocado, vanilla, sweetener and water until creamy. Slowly add in lecithin and blend well. Chill in the fridge for a few minutes, then serve.

2 cups of cashews (soaked or sprouted)
2 green apples, grated
1 to 2 tablespoons of raw honey
½ cup of fresh mint
2 tablespoons of lecithin granules
½ to 1 cup of purified water

green apple, honey & mint whip ...
makes 2 to 3 cups

Blend the cashews, apple, raw honey, mint and purified water until creamy. Slowly add in lecithin and blend well. Chill in the fridge before serving.

fermenting seed and nut yoghurts

Pour yoghurt mix into a glass jar and cover with a cheesecloth. Set in a warm place and allow it to heat up to 90 degrees F Let this sit for 8 to 10 hours, taste for tartness **OR** blend the yoghurt with ½ teaspoon of probiotic powder. The heat from the blender and the probiotic turns the cream into yoghurt

These yummy scrambles are a great alternative to using eggs for breakfast. Even though I love eggs and I definitely recommend these in most diets, some people are allergic to eggs, so in these cases there are still some wonderful breakfast scrambles that can satisfy the taste buds of an egg lover.

breakfast scrambles ...

healthy scrambled 'not eggs'
makes 2 to 3 serves

Blend ingredients together in a processor, adding a little water to get to a nice chunky texture This is a great 'scramble base' to make yummy breakfast scrambles with onions, chilli, shallots mushrooms, tomato and more

- 2 cups of almonds (soaked and/or sprouted)
- 1 cup of sunflower or pumpkin seeds
- ½ teaspoon of Celtic salt
- ½ small onion
- 1 tablespoon of tamari or Bragg's
- 1 tablespoon of fresh grated turmeric (or 1 tsp of turmeric powder)
- ½ lemon, juiced
- a dash of black pepper
- 2 tablespoons of olive oil
- a little purified water

oriental scrambled 'not eggs'
makes 2 small plates

Soak diced bok choy in tamari or Braggs, lime juice and sesame oil. In a blender, pulse healthy scramble mix with rice vinegar, shallots, sesame oil, coriander, red capsicum and marinated bok choy or simply chop ingredients and mix together. Place on two plates and sprinkle black sesame seeds on top with fresh lemon juice

- 1 cup of healthy scrambled 'not eggs' (recipe above)
- ¼ cup of tamari or Braggs
- 2 tablespoons of black sesame seeds
- 2 tablespoons of brown rice vinegar
- ½ cup of shallots or spring onions, diced
- 1 red capsicum, diced
- 3 tablespoons of sesame oil
- a handful of coriander, finely diced
- a handful of bok choy or tat soi, diced

mediterranean scrambled 'not eggs'

makes 2 small plates

1 to 2 cups of healthy scrambled 'not eggs'
1 large red capsicum, diced
½ cup of cherry tomatoes, quartered
½ cup of red or purple onion, finely diced
a handful of fresh basil, shredded
1 cup of baby spinach
2 tablespoons of pure balsamic vinegar
1 lemon, juiced

If you do not have a food processor, place the healthy scramble mix in a bowl and stir through capsicum, tomatoes, basil, baby spinach, red onion, lemon juice and balsamic. If you have a good processor, pulse ingredients and serve on a bed of spinach leaves

mexican scrambled 'not eggs'

makes 2 small plates

1 to 2 cups of healthy scrambled 'not eggs'
1 tomato, finely diced
½ onion, finely diced
1 corn cob, shredded
1 avocado, diced
1 lemon, squeezed
¼ teaspoon of cayenne pepper
¼ teaspoon of paprika
1 jalapeno pepper, finely diced
¼ teaspoon of celtic salt

Use a knife to shred the corn from the cob. Mix the corn with onion, avocado, tomato, jalapeno, lemon juice, cayenne, paprika, salt and healthy scramble mix in a bowl OR place all ingredients in a processor and pulse, keeping slightly chunky. If you are not a fan of spicy foods, leave out the jalapeno and cayenne

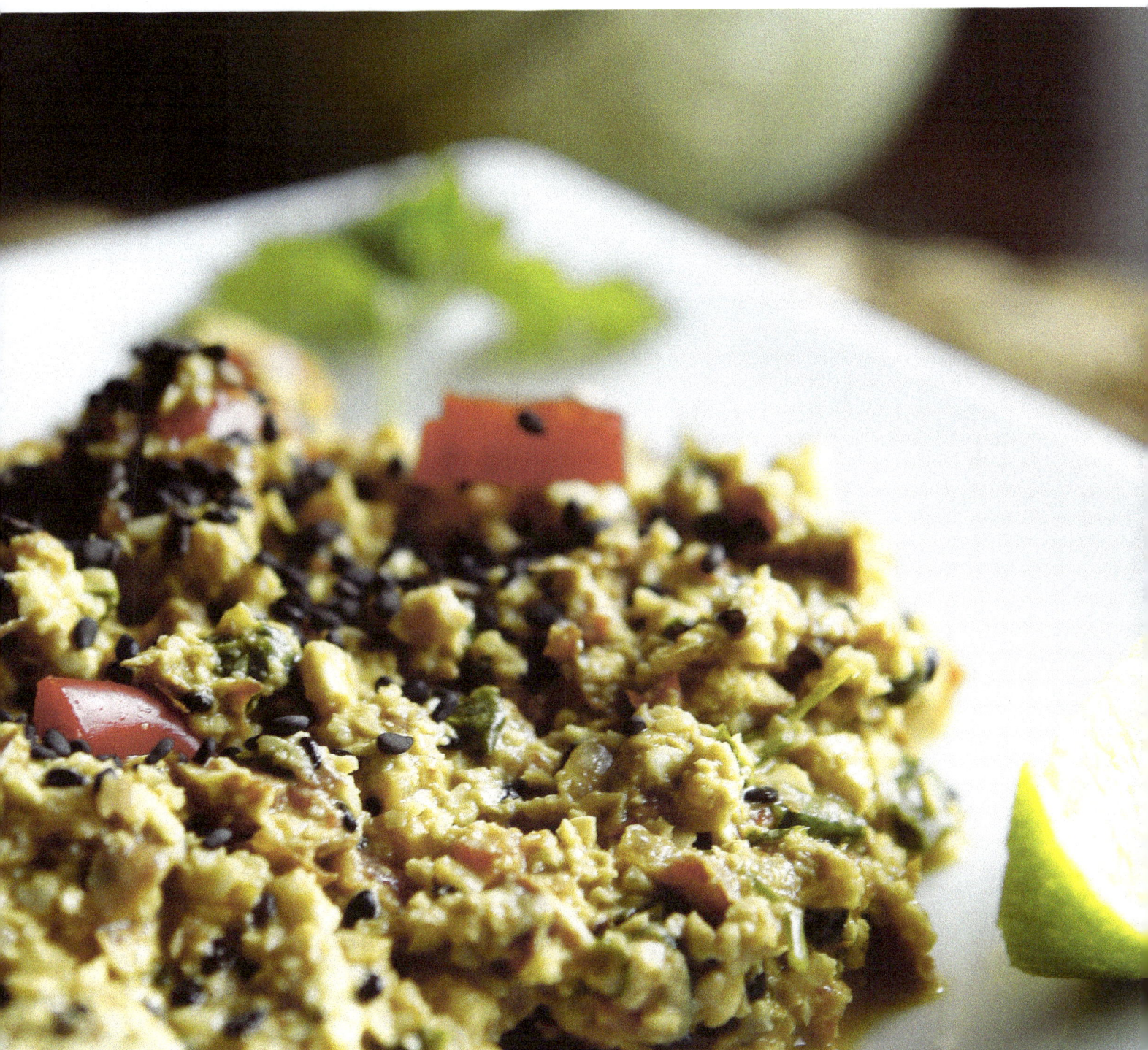

Healthy Breads
Thyme and Olive Bread
Sprouted Essene Bread

Crackers and Chips
Sunny Flaxseed Crackers
Yummy Buckwheat
Spicy Corn Chips
Super Frech Fries
Sun-Dried Tomato and Black Olive Crackers
Sweet Beet Chips
Volcano Chips

Raw Pizza Bases

Breads, Crackers and Chips ...

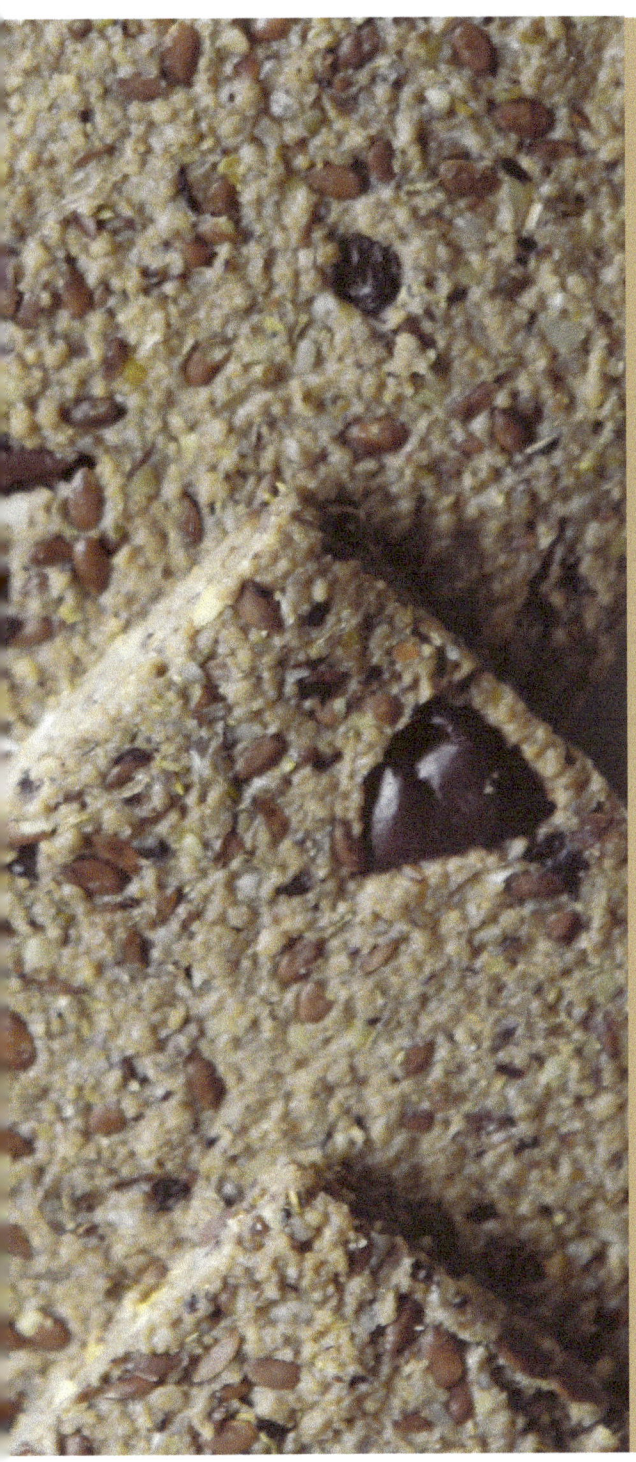

Everyone loves a crusty piece of sourdough toast dipped in steaming hot pumpkin soup on a cold winter's day. While this sounds appetizing, the problem with most of the breads sold today is what they are made of. Many commercial breads, crackers and chips are made from refined vegetable oils high in saturated fats, gluten, preservatives, colourings, additives and huge amounts of sodium. A high of intake of these types of substances can cause weight gain, constipation, fatigue, yeast overgrowth, diverticulitis, heart disease, high blood pressure and even cancer. Most of the breads and crackers found in the supermarkets are made from refined grains that have been stored for long periods of time, making them not only devoid in nutrition but also a major cause of food intolerances.

The healthiest breads are made from sprouted grains like millet, buckwheat, kamut, wheat berries or other grains. When the grain is sprouted, it unlocks the grain's enzyme and nutrient potential making the bread highly nutritious and easy to digest. The crackers, chips and breads in this chapter are made by 'dehydration' to ensure that the enzymes and nutrients are still alive within these foods. Even though I can make some delicious dehydrated snacks I do not do a lot of dehydrating. This is simply because it takes quite a long time to dehydrate foods and with taking care of a family and a full time business I often don't have this time. Also, I love to bite into the crisp flavours, textures and watery content of living foods, something that I do not get from dehydrated snacks. If you do have some spare time and you love breads and crackers, then dehydrated snacks will be great for you. I use a lot of flaxseeds in my dehydrated crackers, breads, chips and pizza bases as they are inexpensive, extremely healthy and I can make lots of different crackers at one time to store and use for later. I have included some of my favourite dehydrated snacks to accompany the yummy dips and spreads found throughout 'Raw Addiction'.

healthy breads ...

thyme and olive bread ...
makes 1 small loaf – 5 to 6 pieces

1 cup of flaxseed meal
½ cup of whole pre-soaked flaxseeds
½ cup of sunflower seeds
½ cup of pumpkin seeds
2 teaspoons of Celtic salt
1 tablespoon of thyme
2 cloves of garlic, minced
½ cup of black olives
¼ to 1 cup of purified water

Soak sunflower seeds, pumpkin seeds and flaxseeds for six hours or overnight. Wash and drain the seeds. Mix ½ cup of soaked flaxseeds with flaxseed meal, other seeds, salt, thyme, garlic and water. Chop olives and knead into the mix. Spread the batter onto teflex sheets and flatten thinly (1/2 to 1 cm thick) with the back of the spatula. Cook at 115 F or 46 C for four to six hours. Score into bread shapes, flip over and dehydrate on a mesh screen on the other side until ready. I love this bread with healthy burgers and garlic aioli.

sprouted essene bread ...
makes 1 loaf

4 cups of sprouted kamut, spelt, rye or wheat berries (refer to sprouting table)
¼ cup of extra virgin olive oil
2 tablespoons of minced garlic
1 tablespoon of caraway seeds
2 teaspoons of Celtic salt
2 to 3 pitted dates (optional)
¼ cup of walnuts or almonds (optional)

To make a simple essene bread, puree all ingredients except for nuts and dates in a food processor until it forms a dough. Spread the mixture onto a teflex sheet and form into the shape of small loaves. Dehydrate at 105 F or 40 C for 13 or more hours. Check with a poker or knife that it is moist on the inside and crispy on the outside. To change the flavour of this bread, add soaked dates and nuts to the mix. You can also swap caraway for another type of seed for variety.

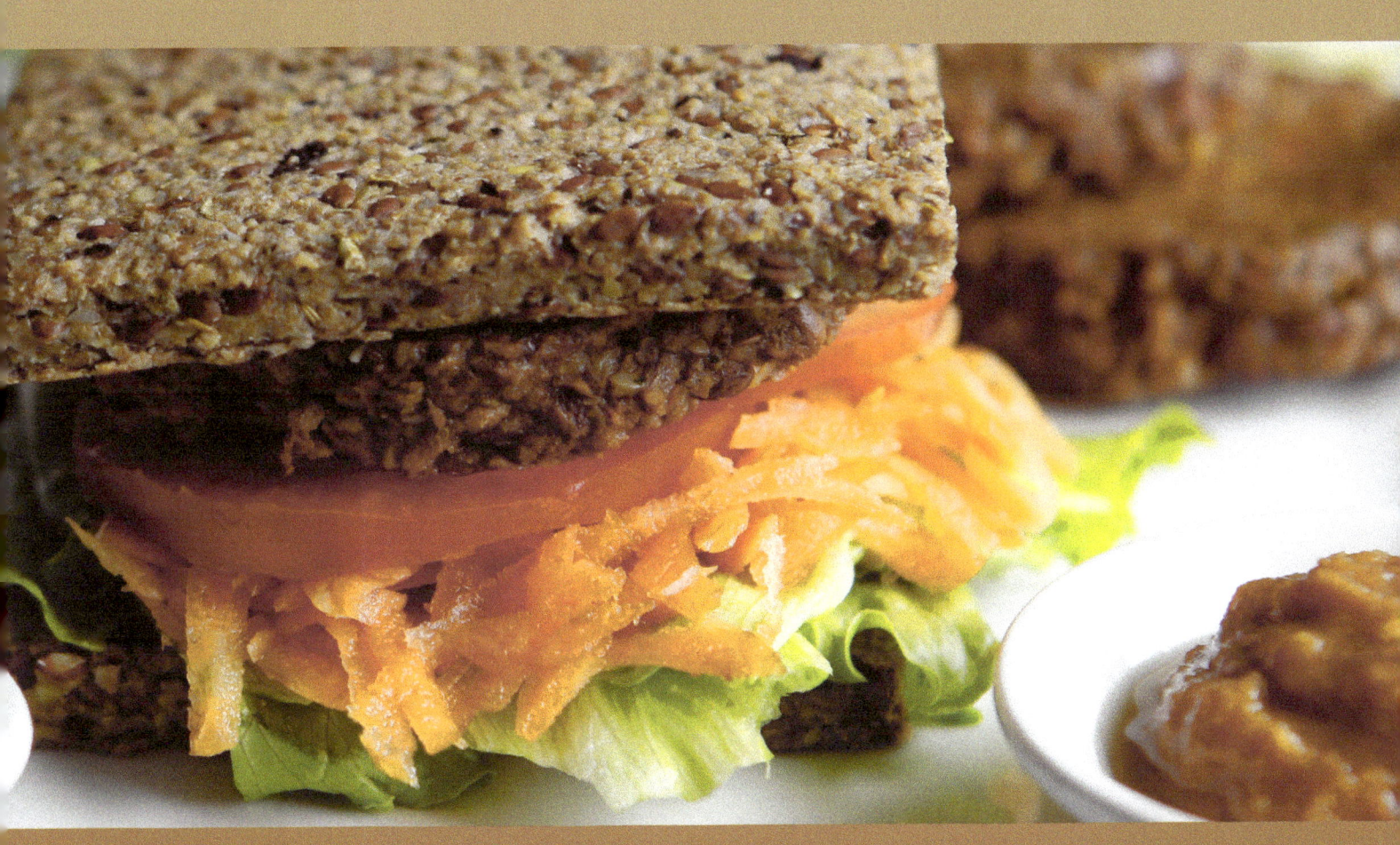

what is ESSENE?

Essene bread is one of the original breads made at least 6000 years ago. 'Essene' is taken from a recipe of the ancient Essenes, a mystic Jewish religious sect that lived in the Middle East around the 1st century. They lived on the Dead Sea and lived by the love of God, virtue, living foods and respect for all life forms. Essene is bread made from sprouted grains. They could make an 'indigestible' grain easy to digest, delicious and full of nutrition.

crackers and chips ...

2 cups of pre-soaked flaxseeds
½ cup of sunflower seeds
½ cup of pumpkin seeds
1 red capsicum
1 small carrot
½ fresh onion
2 garlic cloves
2 teaspoons of Celtic salt
black pepper

sunny flaxseed crackers ...
makes 2 trays of crackers

Soak all seeds overnight. Rinse and add 2 cups of soaked flaxseeds to the rest of the ingredients in a food processor. Blend until it has a nice, doughy texture. Spread thinly on a teflex sheet and dehydrate at 105 F or 40 C until the top is dry, score into the shapes you like, flip over and dehydrate on mesh screens on the other side. When crisp, break into cracker shapes and enjoy.

4 cups of buckwheat groats
2 cups of sunflower seeds
½ cup of sesame seeds
1 carrot
1 small onion, chopped
1 teaspoon of Celtic salt
a dash of black pepper

yummy buckwheat crackers ...
makes 3 trays of crackers

Soak the buckwheat groats and seeds for 5 hours or overnight. Drain and then process with the rest of the ingredients in a food processor. Put the dough mixture onto a teflex sheet and flatten thinly with the back of the spatula. Dehydrate at 115 F or 46 C for 4 hours or until dry on one side. Score into cracker shapes, flip over and place on a mesh screen to finish dehydrating on the other side.

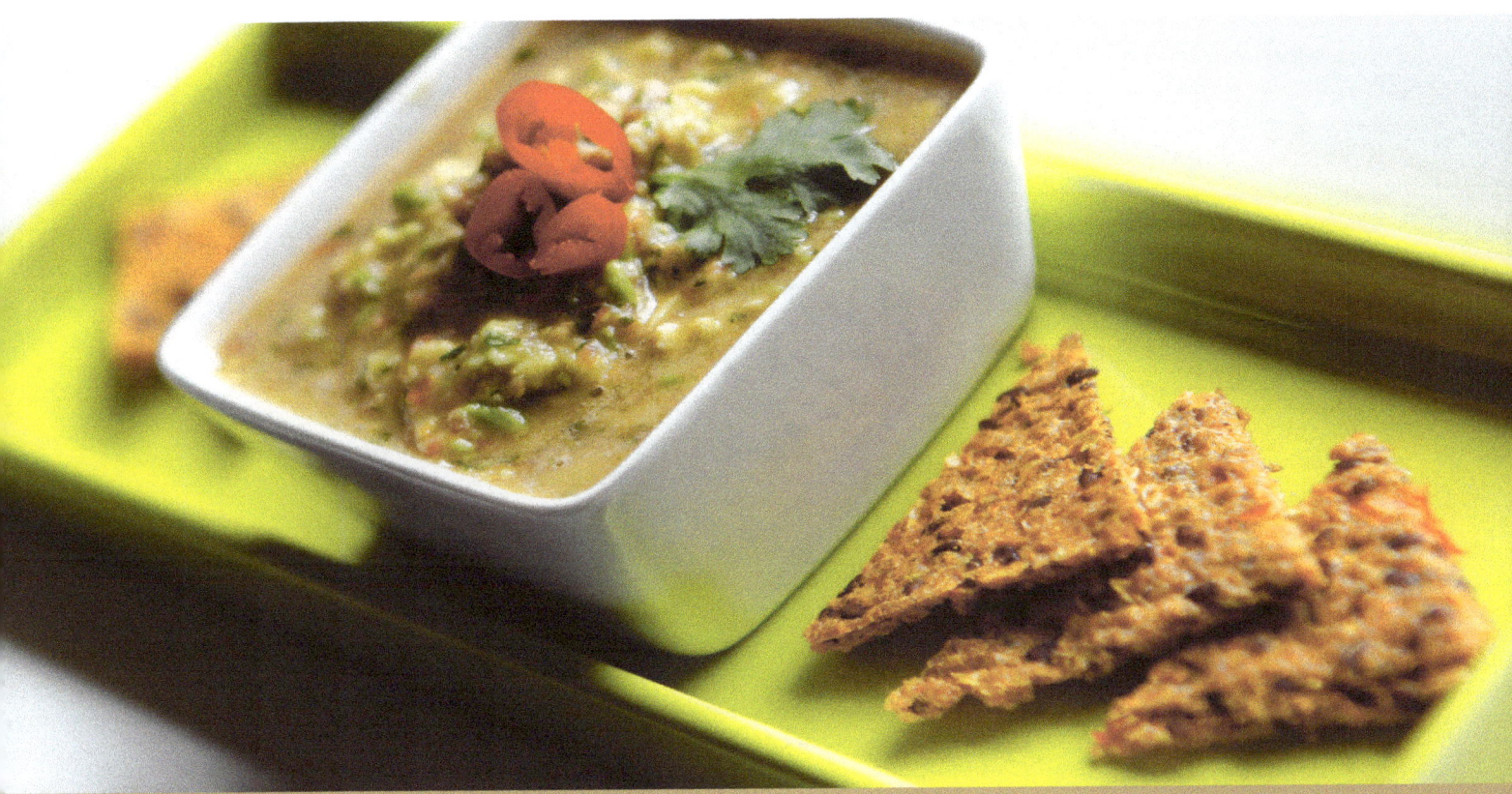

spicy corn chips ...
makes 2 trays of corn chips

3 cobs of corn, fresh
1 cup of flaxseeds (soak overnight and drain well)
½ red pepper, chopped
½ yellow onion, chopped
1 clove of garlic or 1 teaspoon of garlic powder
2 to 3 teaspoons of Celtic salt
1 teaspoon of chilli powder
1 teaspoon of cayenne
4 tablespoons of olive oil

Remove the kernels from the corn and process in a blender until fine, then slowly add the rest of the ingredients. Spread mixture thinly on a teflex sheet and dehydrate at 145 F or 62 C for one hour and then reduce to 105 F or 40 C cooking until crispy on one side. Score into triangle shapes, flip over and dehydrate on the other side until crispy.

nutritional yeast VS yeast foods ...

Many people think nutritional yeast will encourage yeast overgrowth (candida) within the body - this is false. Nutritional yeast is a form of deactivated yeast called 'saccharomyces cerevisiae' made from mixing sugarcane and beet molasses, harvesting, washing and then drying the yeast. It is brimming with B vitamins, protein, fibre, selenium, manganese and Vitamin B12, making it a perfect food source for vegans. It does not feed yeast in the body, as the name suggests, rather it feeds you with valuable nutrition. Nutritional yeast is a perfect addition to use in dehydrated crackers, breads and biscuits.

super french fries

4 cups of sliced swedes, parsnips, sweet potato or any other vegetable
2 teaspoons of turmeric
1 teaspoon of cumin
1 teaspoon of Celtic salt
cold pressed olive oil

Cut the vegetables into French fry or chip shapes. Put olive oil into a bowl with spices. Coat the vegetables with the mix and pat off oil. Place on a teflex sheet and dehydrate at 115 F or 46 C or until golden brown. A brilliant alternative for healthy nachos – without the corn chips.

sun-dried tomato and black olive crackers
makes 2 to 3 trays of crackers

¾ cup of soaked flaxseeds
5 cups of walnuts (soak for 1 to 2 hours)
⅛ cup of nutritional yeast or lecithin granules
3 cups of zucchini, diced
1 cup of sun-dried tomatoes
1 red pepper, chopped
¼ cup of black olives
1 lemon, juiced
1 tablespoon of Celtic salt
purified water

Puree walnuts, olives, zucchini, tomatoes and red pepper. Slowly add in flaxseeds, lemon juice, yeast or lecithin and salt. Add water to make a dough like texture. Spread onto teflex sheets and dehydrate at 115 F or 46 C for six hours, score into cracker shapes, flip over and dehydrate on the other side. Cut into squares and enjoy with dips.

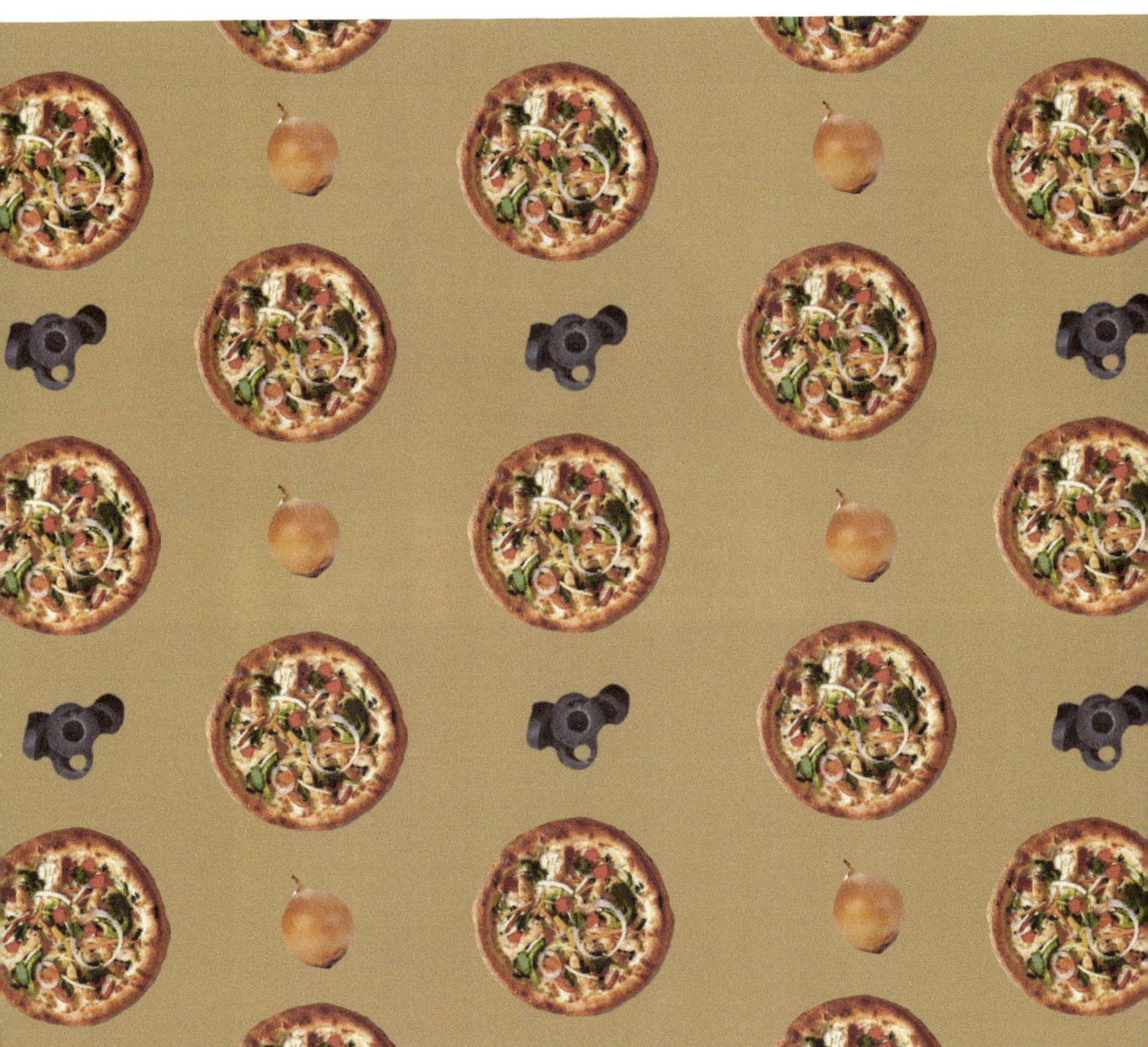

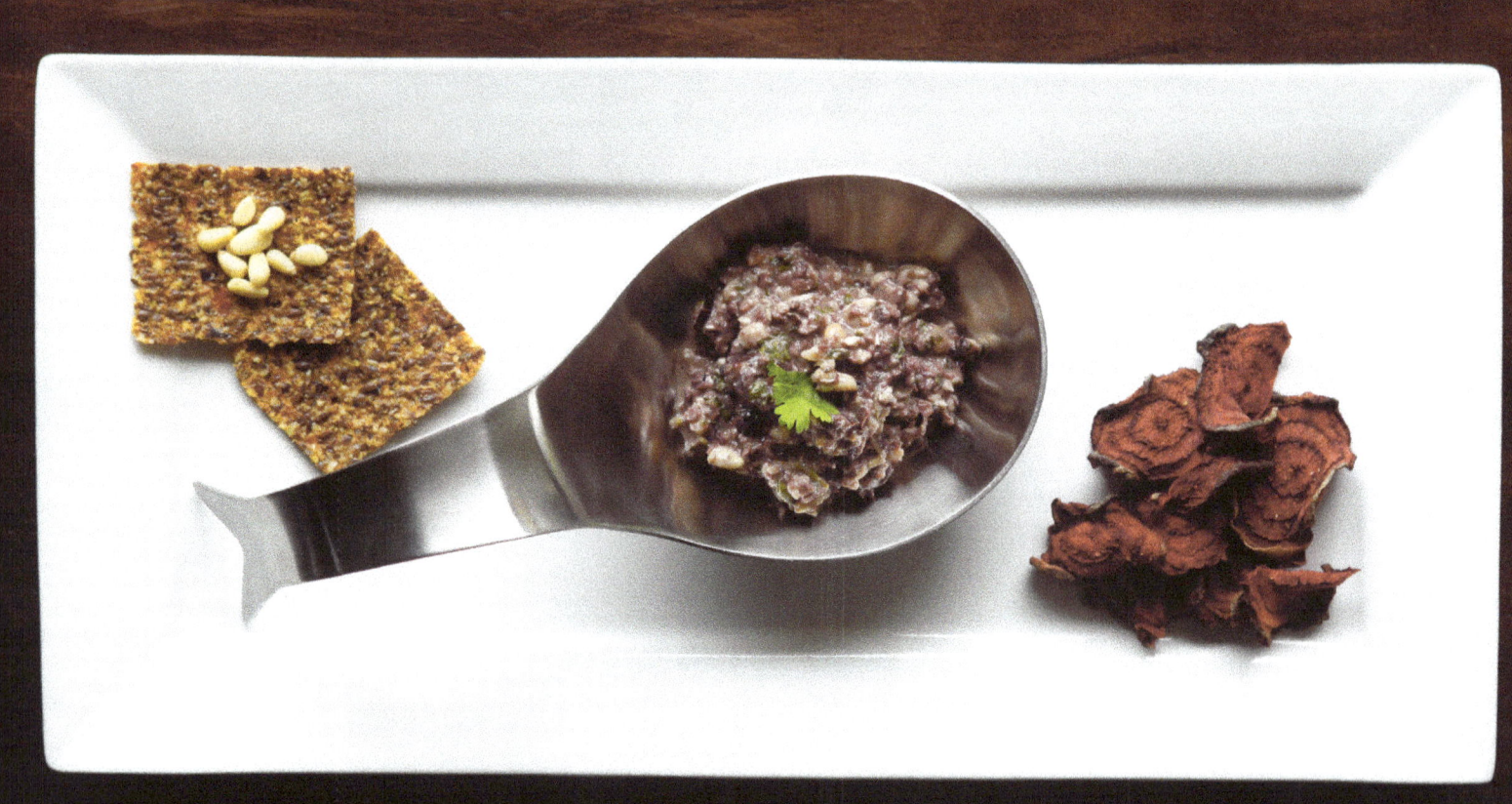

sweet beet chips
makes 3 trays

**3 to 4 whole beets
apple cider vinegar
celtic salt**

These are really easy to make and they taste delicious with all types of dips. Cut the beetroot into very thin slices. Dip or soak in raw apple cider vinegar. Place the chips onto mesh screens, sprinkle with Celtic salt or other yummy spices Dehydrate at a higher heat, 145 F or 62 C for around 1 hour, decrease heat to 115 F or 46 C until crisp and hard

flaxseeds – nature's perfect food ...

I use a lot of flaxseeds in my crackers, chips and breads because they are inexpensive, tasty and contain some amazing healing properties. Flaxseeds are a natural laxative that can sweep the bowel clean of toxins, heavy metals and bad hormones. The high lignan and omega 3 acid content found in this little seed gives great protection against melanoma, colon, breast and prostate cancer. They contain magnesium to boost energy and calm the nerves, omega 3 fats to reduce inflammation and natural phyto-estrogens to prevent menopausal hot flushes. This nutritious seed is 'heart loving' as it can guard against high blood pressure, high cholesterol and atherosclerosis. If you want to lose weight, don't forget to add flaxseeds to your weight loss program.

volcano chips ...
makes 2 trays of chips

1 cup of sunflower seeds
1 cup of walnuts
1 cup of almonds
1 cup of chopped tomato
1 red capsicum, chopped
2 garlic cloves
1 teaspoon of Celtic salt
1 teaspoon of cayenne
1 teaspoon of paprika
1 teaspoon of chilli powder
2 to 4 tablespoons of olive oil
a little purified water

Soak nuts for 4 to 5 hours or overnight. Drain and puree with the rest of the ingredients in a food processor. Spread thinly onto teflex sheets and dehydrate at 115 F or 46 C for four hours or until dry on one side. Score into chip shapes, flip over and cook on a mesh screen on the other side until ready.

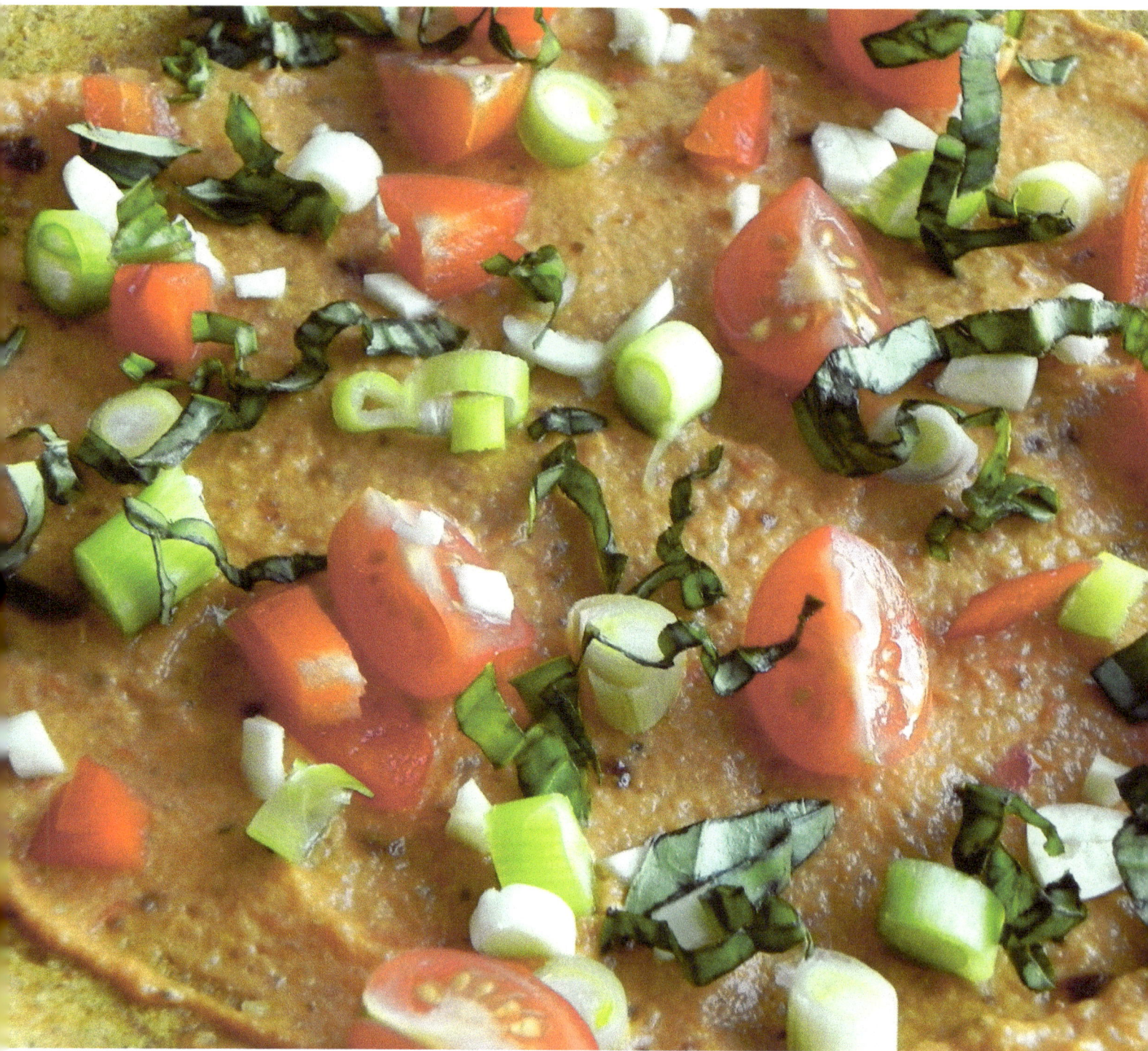

raw pizza base 1 ...
makes 2 large pizza bases or 4 small ones

2 cups of buckwheat groats (sprouted or soaked) or soaked flaxseeds
4 tablespoons of olive oil
3 celery stalks
1 carrot, chopped
⅛ onion or 2 spring onions
2 garlic cloves
2 teaspoons of celtic salt

Soak buckwheat groats or flaxseeds overnight. Use 2 cups of soaked flaxseeds or buckwheat groats and puree with the rest of the ingredients. Oil up a teflex sheet and spread dough thinly onto this. Press into pizza shapes. Dehydrate at 115 F or 46 C for 3 to 4 hours or until dry on one side, flip over and put back onto a mesh screen to dehydrate on the other side until ready.

raw pizza base 2 ...
makes 2 large pizza bases or 4 small ones

1 cup of almonds (pre-soaked)
1 cup of soaked flaxseeds
¼ cup of sun-dried tomatoes
¼ cup of chopped tomatoes or cherry tomatoes
2 tablespoons of olive oil
2 tablespoons of lecithin granules or nutritional yeast
2 teaspoons of celtic salt

Pre-soak almonds and flaxseeds overnight. Use 1 cup of the soaked flaxseeds and 1 cup of soaked almonds and puree with tomatoes, olive oil, yeast or lecithin and celtic salt. Put a little oil onto a teflex sheet and spread dough mixture into pizza shapes very thinly. Dehydrate at 115 F or 46 C for 4 hours or until dry on one side. Flip over, place on a mesh screen and dehydrate on the other side until ready.

Fantastic Fillings
Nutty Meat

Scrumptious Sauces and Spreads
Almond Butter
Organic Almond Mayo
Spicy Cauliflower Mayo
Tomato Ketchup
Simple Mayo
Garlic Cashew Aioli
Spicy Gravy

Delicious Dips
Natural Dippers
Pistachio and Turmeric Dip
Traditional Guacamole
Asian Guacamole
Spicy Tomato Salsa
Vegetable Hummus
Wasabi Mayonnaise
Olive and Coriander Tapenade
Basic Pesto
Macadamia Pesto
Roasted Baba Ganoush
Brazilian Goji Berry Salsa
Spicy Miso Dip
Spinach and Coriander Dip

Mock Cheese
Tex Mex
Crunchy Garlic Parmesan
Basic 'Mock Cheese'
Pizza Pete
Macho Nacho

Salad Dressings
Spring Miso
Tahini Treat
Siam Sunrise
Asian Creation
Sweet Beet
Black Sesame
Garlic Tahini
Sweet Mustard
Red Volcano
Hot Sombrero
Ginger and Sesame
Cool Mint
Sunny Carrot
Red Capsicum and Chilli

Superb Spreads, Dips and Condiments …

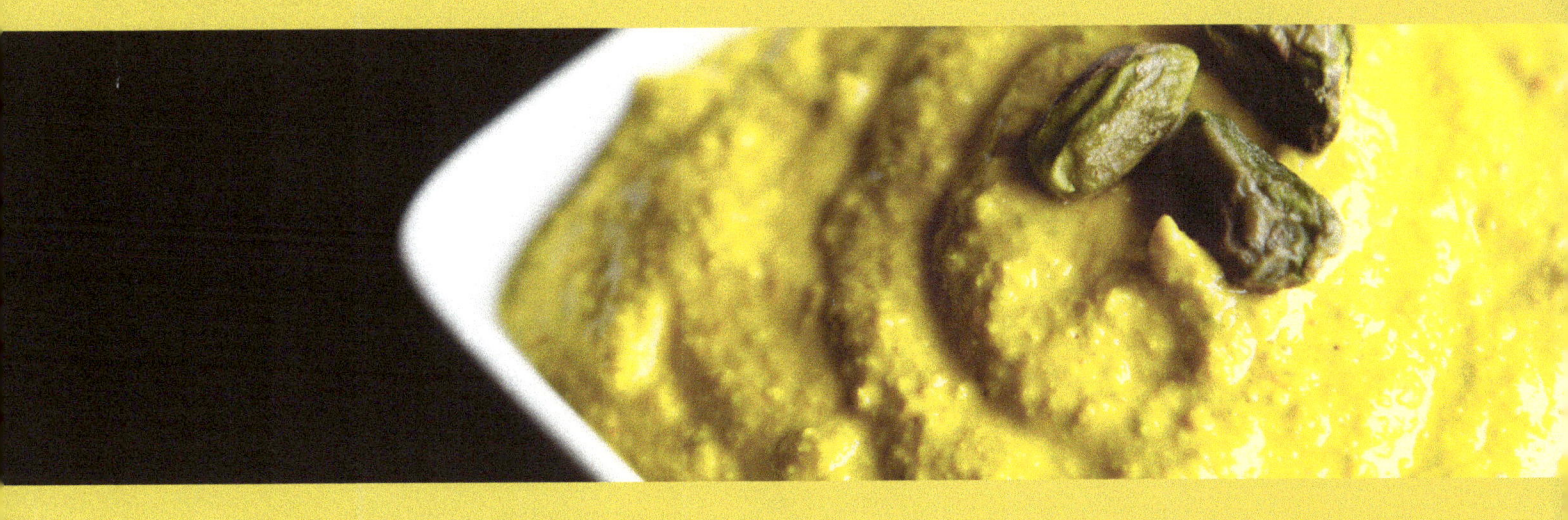

fantastic fillings ...

nutty meat

makes 1 bowl of nutty meat

⅛ cup of almonds
¼ cup of sunflower or pumpkin seeds
⅛ teaspoon of ground cumin
⅛ teaspoon of turmeric
¼ fresh onion or 1 tablespoon of onion powder
¼ cup of extra virgin olive or flaxseed oil
1 teaspoon of celtic salt
2 tablespoon of tamari or Braggs
a dash of paprika or cayenne
1/3 cup of fresh mint, basil or coriander (change for different flavours)
3 pitted medjool dates (optional)
a dash of black pepper
purified water

Blend almonds and seeds with cumin, turmeric, oil, onion, salt, tamari or braggs, herbs and enough purified water to make a thick mix. This stores for four to five days in the fridge

Nutty meat is the perfect vegetarian alternative for meat lovers, especially if you feel like something more savoury and filling. It is full of healthy monounsaturated fats to beautify the skin and protect against cardiovascular disease and cancer. When I feel like a satisfying snack, I wrap some nutty meat in lettuce or cabbage leaves and devour. The beauty of this nutty meat is you can change the flavour by swapping the herbs and spices used. Nutty meat is also perfect in lettuce or cabbage burrito's or taco cups with Asian guacamole, macho nacho cheese and salsa. Absolutely delicious!!!

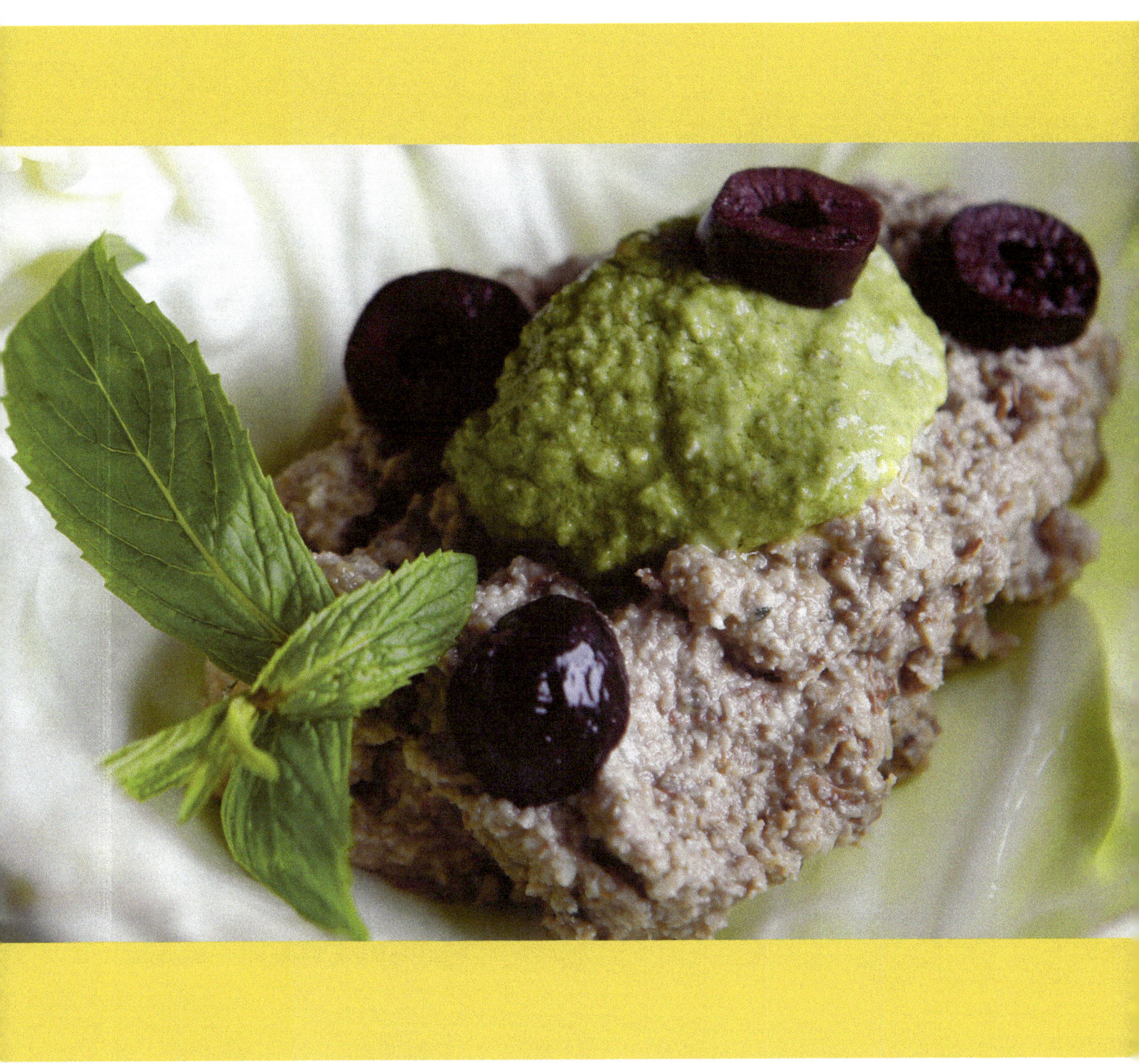

almond butter

makes 1 jar of almond butter

2 cups of almonds
(pre-soaked for 5 to 6 hours)
½ cup of purified water

Drain almonds and add to the food processor with liquid. Use as little of the water as possible to get a thicker mix. If you want this even thicker, blend almonds with nut milk. Place in a jar and store in the fridge. This will last for at least five days in the fridge when opened

scrumptious sauces and spreads ...

organic almond mayonnaise

makes 1 tub of mayonnaise

1 cup of almonds
(pre-soaked to soften)
1 lemon, juiced
1 tablespoon of raw apple cider vinegar
1 garlic clove or 1 tablespoon of minced garlic
3 pitted medjool dates
or 1 tsp of raw agave nectar, stevia or xylitol
3 tablespoons of flaxseed or olive oil
1 teaspoon of celtic salt
1 teaspoon of pure mustard paste, powder or seeds
2 tablespoons of lecithin granules
a few basil leaves
¼ cup of purified water

Blend all of the ingredients (except the oil) until smooth. Now begin to add the oil and slowly blend. Place in a glass jar and refrigerate for a few hours to let this set. This is a very delicious, nutty tasting mayonnaise that is low in saturated fat, yet high in healthy monounsaturated fats

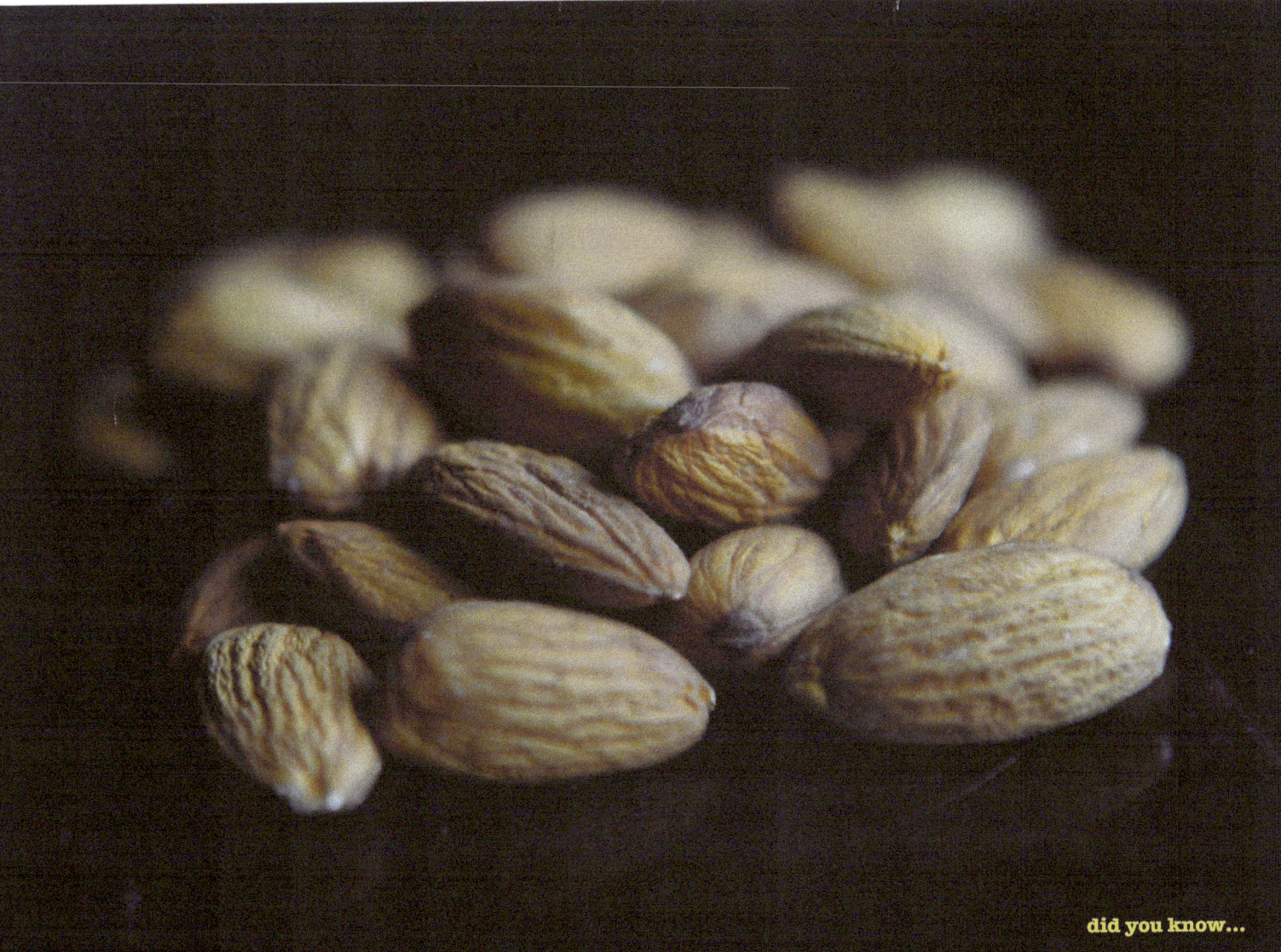

did you know…

Almonds are one of the most nutritious nuts found on the planet. They contain huge amounts of healthy mono-unsaturated fats. These fats lower bad cholesterol, thereby preventing heart disease. They are full of manganese to steady the nerves and Vitamin E to protect against several forms of cancer. Almonds are not fattening, as most people think. The minerals and healthy fats found in this nut encourage fat burning and weight loss. To top this off, almonds contain a potent cancer fighting substance known as laetrile. So next time you are looking for a simple addition to lose weight and to ward off disease – think of the understated power of the almond

spicy cauliflower mayo
makes 1 tub of mayonnaise

2 cups of fresh cauliflower florets
1 teaspoon of celtic salt
½ teaspoon of organic mustard paste, powder or seeds
¼ teaspoon of turmeric powder
a dash of paprika
a dash of cumin
2 tablespoons of lecithin granules
2 tablespoons of flaxseed or Udo's oil
2 tablespoons of apple cider vinegar
½ lemon, squeezed
a little purified water (for the right consistency)

Put all of the ingredients into a food processor and blend until creamy
Add water to get the perfect texture
A perfect healthy alternative to artery-clogging mayonnaise

cauliflower – the white guardian ...

Cauliflower, the white sister of broccoli, is an incredible body detoxifier, cancer protection agent and anti-inflammatory. It contains huge amounts of Vitamin C to ward off disease, Vitamin K to aid blood clotting, Vitamin B6 to prevent PMS and manganese to steady the nerves. Like broccoli, cauliflower contains glucosinolates. These substances help to detoxify dangerous toxins and hormones that can cause bladder, breast, colon, prostate and ovarian cancer. This understated vegetable is also great for digestion. It contains sulforaphane, a substance which prevents the overgrowth of the Helicobacter pylori bacteria, the major cause of ulcers. Researchers are now revealing its benefit in the treatment of Crohn's, ulcerative colitis and other inflammatory bowel diseases. Wow – what an under-estimated vegetable!

vegetable sunscreen ...

Tomatoes contain a powerful flavonoid called lycopene. Lycopene guards against stomach, prostate, bladder, colon, lung, pancreatic and skin cancer. By eating lots of cooked tomatoes rich in lycopene you can give yourself three times greater sun protection factor. No wonder Mediterranean people have such beautiful skin that never seems to burn. It must be all of the tomatoes from their pasta and pizza dishes. What a yummy way to protect against sun damage.

tomato ketchup ...
makes 1 tub of ketchup

4 fresh tomatoes
(look for ripe roma tomatoes)
½ to 1 cup of sun-dried tomatoes
3 cloves of garlic
4 organic medjool dates, pitted
(or 1 tbsp of yacon syrup, stevia or other)
1 tablespoon of tamari
¼ cup of apple cider vinegar
a handful of fresh basil leaves
1 teaspoon of Celtic salt
a little purified water

Put all ingredients into a blender or processor and puree. This is a yummy tomato sauce that can be used as the base for a vegetable pasta, on raw pizza bases, or as tomato ketchup (simply by adding more water). To get a sweeter ketchup, use roma or cherry tomatoes. To make runnier, add more purified water.

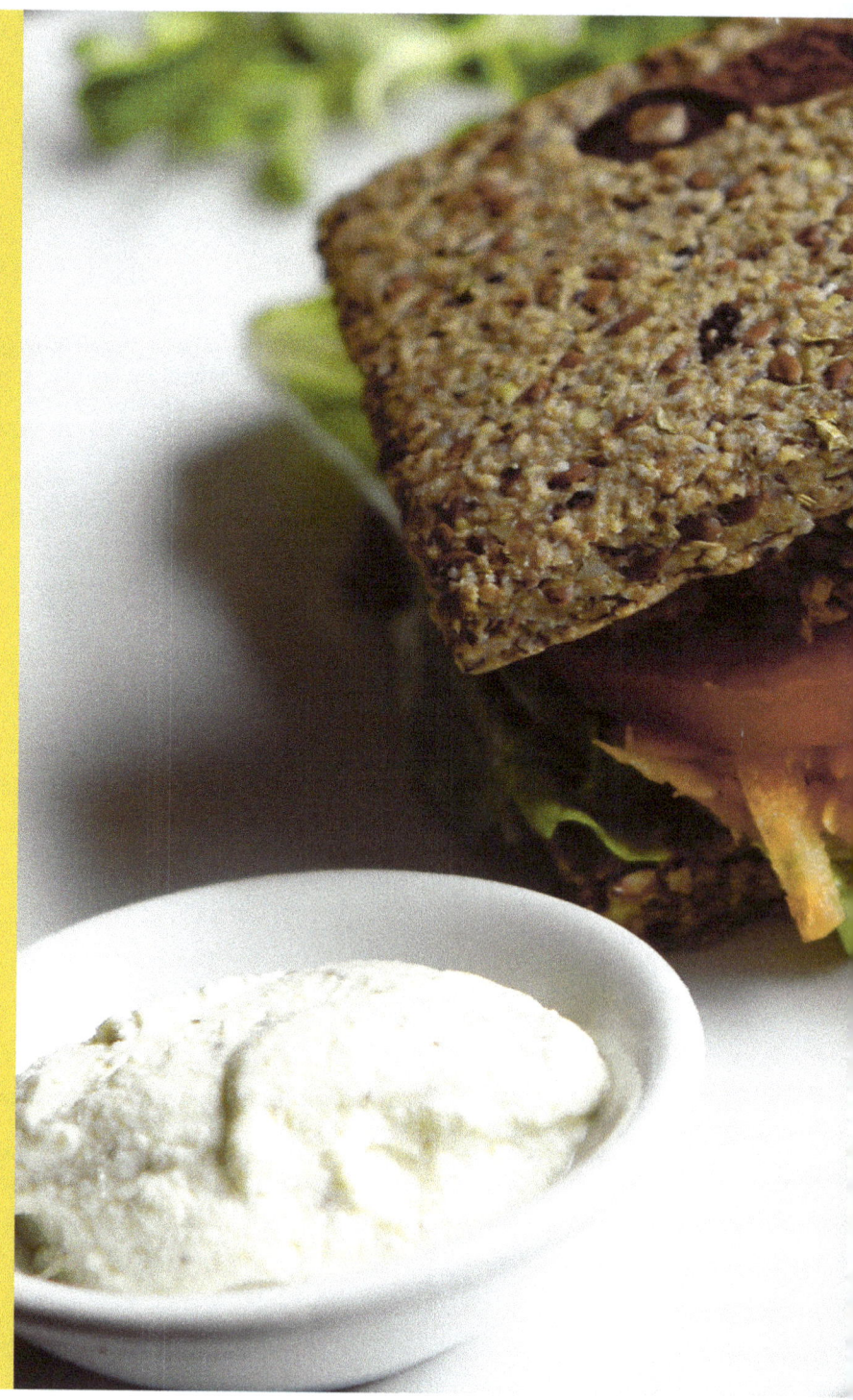

simple mayo
makes 1 tub of mayo

1 cup of cashews (pre-soaked to soften)
¼ cup of fresh lemon juice
¼ cup of tomato, chopped
2 garlic cloves
2 tablespoons of lecithin granules
3 tablespoons of olive or flaxseed oil
a little purified water
a dash of celtic salt
a small handful of fresh parsley

Combine all ingredients in a food processor and blend until creamy. If you use roma tomatoes it will have a sweeter taste. If you want to thicken the mayo, add more lecithin granules and cashews. This keeps for around three to five days when refrigerated

nature's antibiotic …

Garlic is often referred to as 'nature's antibiotic' as it stands guard against all types of viruses, bacteria, microbes and parasites. It has proven itself a worthy immune warrior and cancer protection agent in thousands of worldwide studies. It is a heart smart herb that lowers cholesterol and blood pressure guarding against blood clots, strokes and heart attacks. Garlic is a wonderful source of germanium, an antioxidant that supersaturates the body's cells with oxygen. No wonder I include garlic in so many recipes.

1 cup of organic cashews
(pre-soaked for 3 to 5 hours)
1 lemon, juiced
1 celery stalk
2 tablespoons of fresh or dried thyme
3 garlic cloves
1 teaspoon of Celtic salt
1 tablespoon of raw apple cider vinegar
1 teaspoon of cumin
¼ cup of water

garlic cashew aioli …
makes 1 bottle of aioli

Blend all of the ingredients until creamy.
If you don't want this aioli too spicy, use a little less garlic.

1 tablespoon of pure miso paste
(shiro or genmai)
1 tablespoon of red wine vinegar
1 small onion, chopped
1 clove of garlic (or 1 tsp of minced garlic)
¼ cup of purified water or carrot juice
¼ cup of organic sesame oil
1 small red chilli
(or 1 to 2 teaspoons of red chilli paste)
1 tablespoon of tamari or Bragg's
2 medjool dates, pitted
1 lime, squeezed

spicy gravy …
makes 1 cup of spicy gravy

Combine all ingredients in a processor and blend until runny. This is my favourite gravy that I love to pour over everything, especially dehydrated vegetable chips and salads. This keeps for around 3 days in the fridge.

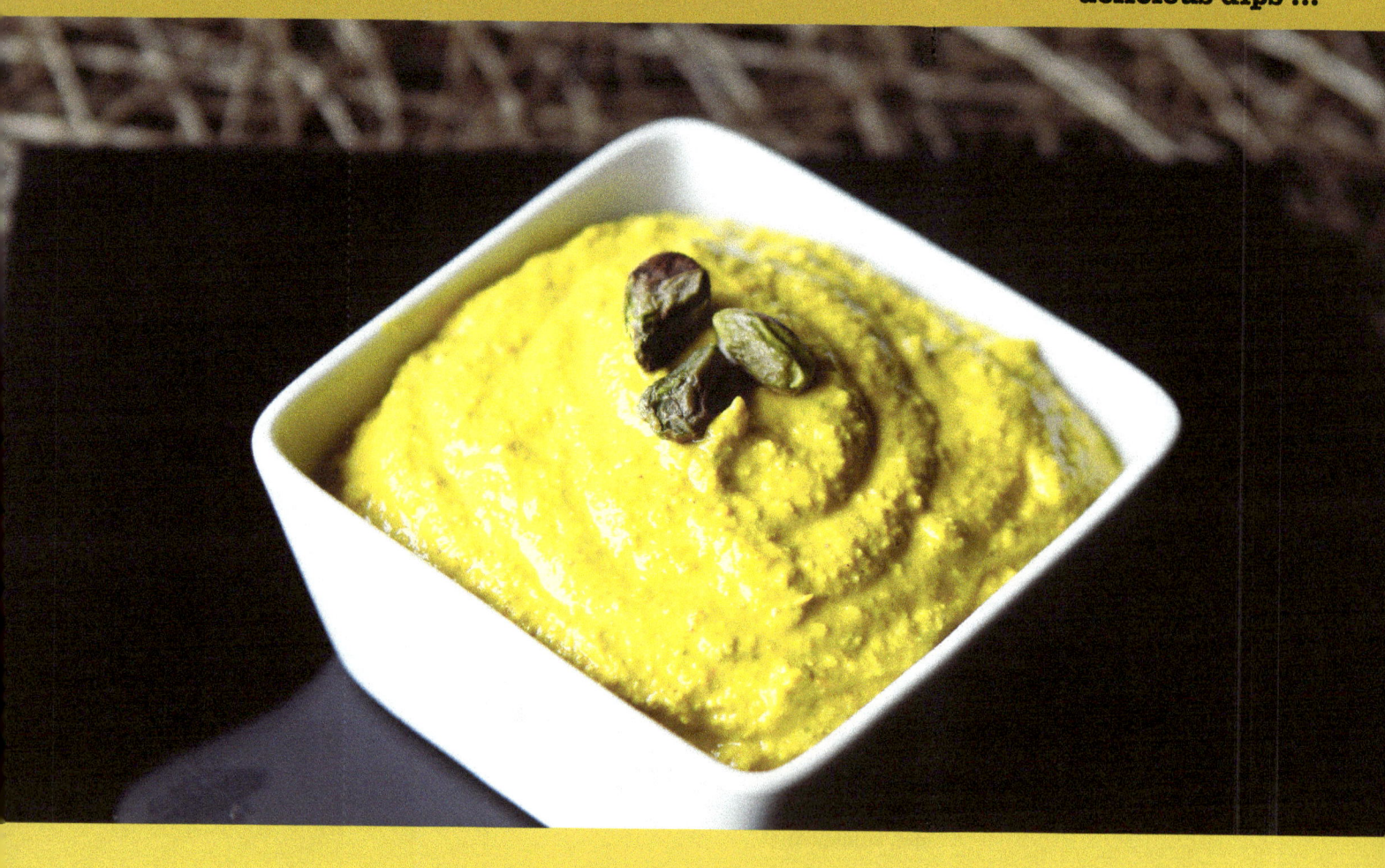

delicious dips …

natural dippers ...

Everyone loves a crispy, crunchy chip or cracker to use with soups or dips. Most packaged chips are made with unhealthy trans fats that clog up arteries and cause diabetes, heart disease and even cancer. But luckily there are some healthy options available. My favourite natural dippers are:

raw veggie sticks ...
Try using carrots, zucchini, celery, cucumber, asparagus, red, orange or green capsicum and more....

crunchy veggie chips ...
Cut up any vegetable, sprinkle with a little olive oil, tamari & celtic salt and cook in a dehydrator or oven until crunchy.

natural sweet potato chips ...
Peel and slice sweet potatoes, pumpkin, taro or parsnip into very thin slices. Mix in a bowl with celtic salt, tamari, a little olive oil and herbs of your choice, depending on which taste you like. Personally I love sweet potato chips with cayenne and paprika. Place on a teflex sheet on a dehydrator tray and heat until golden brown, then flip over and heat on the other side.

pistachio and turmeric dip
makes 1 big bowl

Blend all ingredients until creamy in a processor. If you want this dip sweeter, you can add a few organic pitted dates. This is definitely one of my favourite dips. It is full of powerful cancer-fighting and heart-protecting antioxidants and anti-inflammatory agents. This dip guards against cancer, rheumatism, arthritis, heart disease, strokes, high blood pressure and more ...

1 tablespoon of fresh turmeric or turmeric powder
4 tablespoons of hemp seed or flaxseed oil
¼ cup of pistachio nuts
2 garlic cloves
1 teaspoon of cumin
1 to 2 tablespoons of tamari
¼ cup of cherry tomatoes
1 lemon, juiced
a dash of black pepper
a small handful of parsley
a little purified water

traditional guacamole ...
makes 1 bowl

2 to 3 ripe avocados
2 teaspoons of jalapeno (minced or diced)
½ cup of chopped roma tomato
2 teaspoons of Celtic salt
2 fresh lemons, juiced
2 tablespoons of flaxseed or olive oil
¼ purple onion (optional)

Mash avocado and flaxseed oil with a spoon until creamy. Fold in onions, jalapeno, tomato, Celtic salt and lemon juice. This makes a delicious, chunky avocado dip. If you want a smoother guacamole, process ingredients in a blender.

botox in a bowl ...

Avocados are nature's answer to botox. They contain all of the famous skin beautifying ingredients including monounsaturated fats, vitamin A, C, E, D, potassium, lecithin and chlorophyll. These nutrients are famous for their anti-ageing and skin-regenerating properties. The high amount of Vitamin C found in this little fruit is needed for the production of collagen and the growth of new skin cells. And if you are worried about the old myth that avocados are fattening – then don't. Avocados are actually brilliant for weight loss due to their rich levels of oleic acid.

asian guacamole ...
makes one large bowl

2 avocados
2 garlic cloves
1 tablespoon of grated ginger
¼ cup of red cherry tomatoes
1 teaspoon of miso (shiro or genmai)
2 lemons, juiced
¼ cup of coriander
1 red chilli or (1 tsp of minced red chilli)
a dash of Celtic salt

Mash avocado and set aside. In a processor blend the rest of the ingredients and stir into the avocado mix. For extra spice add a little minced red chilli paste with a dash of cayenne pepper. This is not your normal guacamole, but rather a spicy version that also packs a huge nutrient punch in the cancer-fighting arena. Ginger, cayenne and chilli peppers are fantastic circulatory stimulants that contain some powerful anti-cancer ingredients. They are also brilliant for burning stubborn tummy fat.

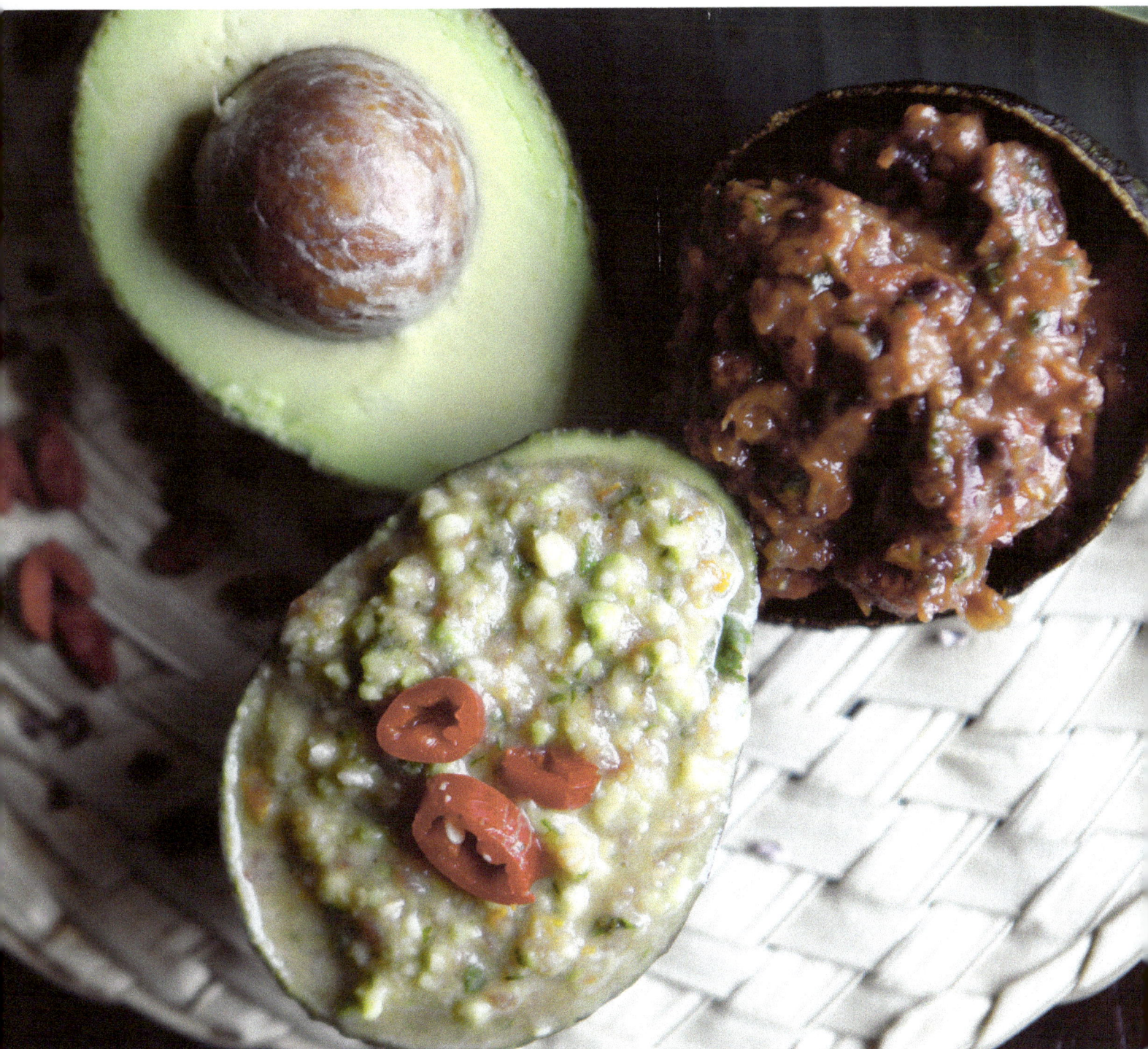

spicy tomato salsa
makes 1 bowl

Place all ingredients in a food processor and pulse quickly. Keep the mixture chunky otherwise it won't be a salsa anymore. I absolutely love this with dehydrated corn chips and chunky guacamole. A yummy, healthy snack

4 ripe romaine tomatoes, diced
2 garlic cloves, diced
4 tablespoons of flaxseed or macadamia oil
2 lemons, squeezed
1 teaspoon of Celtic salt
1 small purple onion, chopped
1 small red bird chilli (or 2 tsp of chilli paste)
1 teaspoon of grated or minced ginger
2 to 3 pitted medjool dates
a handful of coriander

vegetable hummus
makes 1 bowl

In a food processor blend zucchini, olives, tahini, garlic, lemon juice, Celtic salt, paprika and oil until creamy. If you want a sweeter dip, blend in sun-dried tomatoes

2 zucchini, skinned
¼ cup of pitted black olives
¼ cup of tahini
3 garlic cloves
2 lemons, juiced
1 teaspoon of Celtic salt
½ teaspoon of paprika
¼ cup of hemp, udo's or flaxseed oil
1/3 cup of sun-dried tomatoes (optional)

wasabi mayonnaise
makes 1 bottle of mayonnais

Blend all ingredients in a food processor adding water to get a smooth texture. If you love hot and spicy foods like me, add extra wasabi paste. If you don't eat soy, replace tofu with 1 cup of almonds or cashews

½ block of organic tofu or
½ cup of organic pre-soaked cashews
¼ cup of olive or flaxseed oil
2 to 3 garlic cloves
3 teaspoons of wasabi paste or powder
(or pure horseradish paste)
2 teaspoons of mustard paste, powder or seeds
1 teaspoon of celtic salt
4 to 6 tablespoons of apple cider vinegar
3 pitted medjool dates

1 cup of black or green olives
(naturally dried and pitted)
1 to 2 fresh lemons, juiced
3 tablespoons of olive oil
⅓ cup of coriander
2 garlic cloves
¼ cup of pine nuts
lots of fresh cracked pepper

olive and coriander tapenade ...
makes 1 bowl

Pulse all of the ingredients together in a blender – keep slightly chunky. A yummy tapenade to use with vegie sticks or raw crackers and a perfect solution for a 'raw food' dinner party. I love this with 'sweet beet chips'.

appetite suppressant seeds ...

Pine nuts are an amazing weight loss seed. They contain pinolenic acid, a magical essential fatty acid that can trigger the action of hunger suppressing enzymes in the gut, calming down a voracious appetite. Pine nuts also contain good amounts of oleic acid to lower triglycerides and the 'bad cholesterol' that causes heart disease. If you need a B vitamin boost, these are perfect as they contain B1, B2, B3, B5, B6 and folate. To add to their nutritional arsenal, pine nuts are also a superb source of iron, manganese, magnesium, calcium, zinc, and selenium. No wonder I eat so many pine nuts!

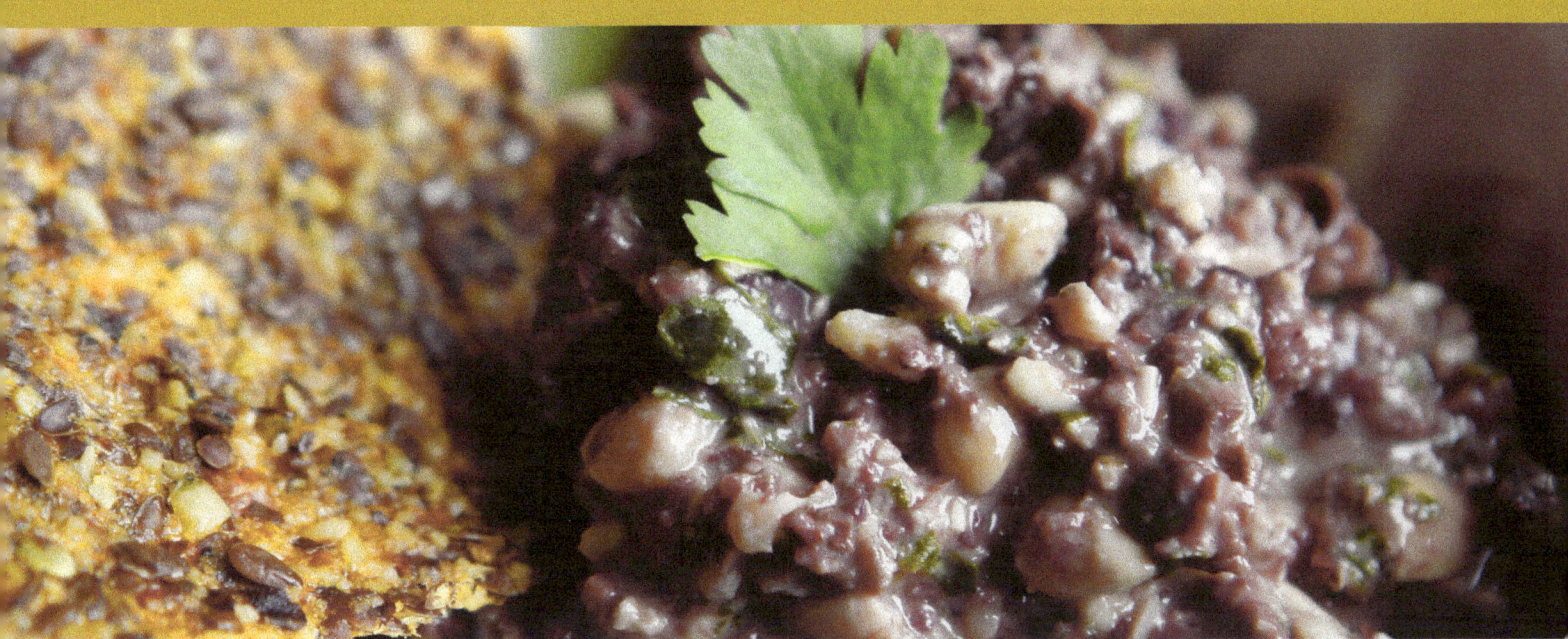

basic pesto
makes 1 cup of pesto

Blend all of the ingredients in a food processor. If you want this runnier, add more lemon juice. If you want this creamier, add more nuts

- ⅛ a bunch of fresh basil
- 1 cup of pine nuts or cashews
- 2 garlic cloves
  (add more if you want spicy)
- 1/3 cup of olive or flaxseed oil
- 1 large lemon, juiced
- 1 tablespoon of tahini
- a large pinch of Celtic salt

macadamia pesto
makes 1 cup of pesto

Process garlic, salt and macadamia nuts into a powder and put aside. Pulse the basil with lemon juice. Add macadamia mix back into the processor with olive oil and blend until creamy. If you want a stronger garlic flavour, add an extra clove of garlic. For a thinner pesto, use one cup of nuts and for a thicker pesto use two cups of nuts

- 2 to 3 cups of basil leaves
- 1 cup of rocket
- 1 cup of baby spinach leaves
- 2 garlic cloves
- 1 to 2 cups of macadamia nuts
- 2 large lemons, juiced
- 1 tablespoon of tahini
- ½ cup of extra virgin olive oil
- a large pinch of Celtic salt

roasted baba ganoush
makes 1 bowl

Cut the eggplant into thin slices, brush with a little olive oil and Celtic salt and dehydrate until golden brown. If you don't have a dehydrator, place under a grill and cook at a low heat until ready. Place eggplant into a processor with the rest of the ingredients and blend until slightly chunky

- 2 eggplants – cut into thin slices
- 2 tablespoons of parsley, chopped
- 3 garlic cloves
- 2 lemons, juiced
- 6 tablespoons of olive oil
- 1 tablespoon of tahini
- ½ teaspoon of cumin
- ½ teaspoon of paprika
- ½ teaspoon of Celtic salt
- ½ teaspoon of cayenne

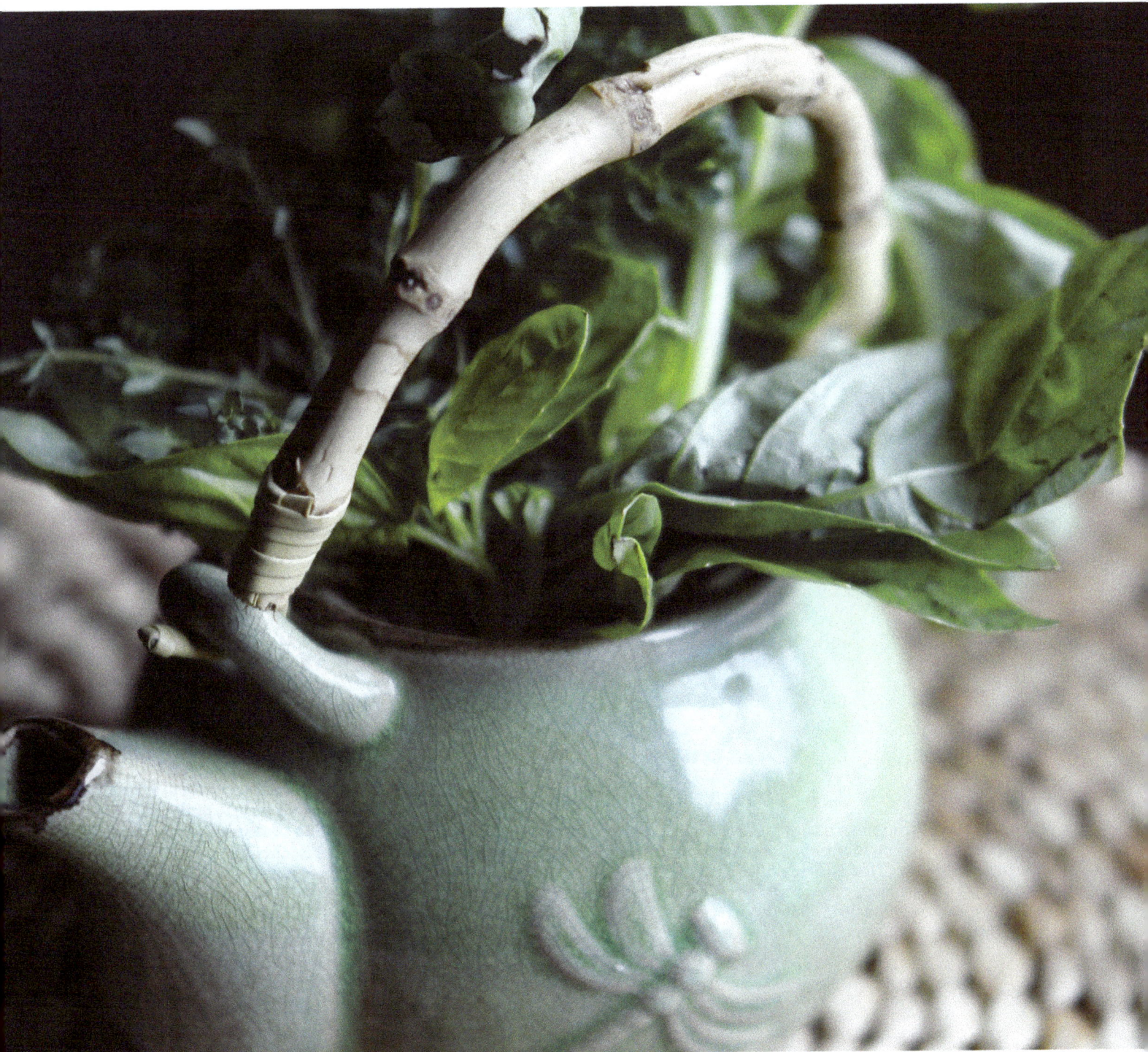

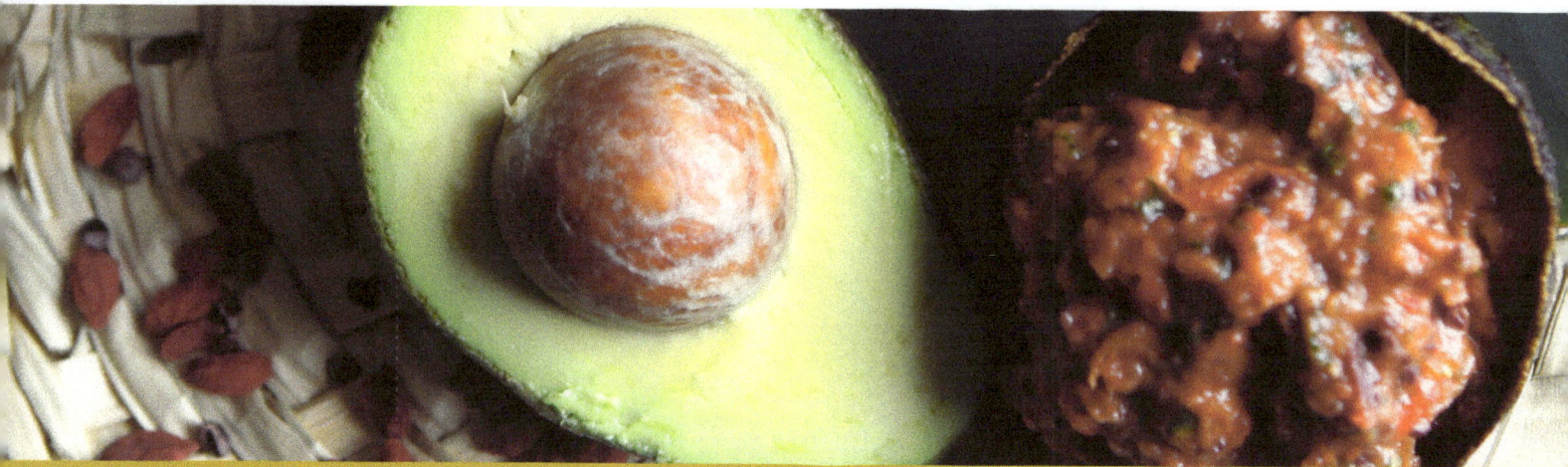

the happy berry ...

Goji berries or Himalayan wolfberries are found in the beautiful Tibetan, Mongolian and Chinese regions of Asia. The Tibetans nicknamed the goji – 'happy berry' because of its ability to evoke happiness and serenity when eaten. Practitioners from these regions have used the goji as a medicine for over 6000 years. Goji berries contain some powerful antioxidants including lutein, beta-carotene and zeaxanthin. These carotenoids are famous for protecting the eyes against macular degeneration. Many test tube studies have proven the benefits of goji in preventing cancer, diabetes and cholesterol problems. This little happy berry powerfully boosts energy and vitality.

brazilian goji berry salsa
makes 1 bowl

Put all of the ingredients into a processor (except for avocado) and pulse the mix, leaving chunky. Chop avocado into small squares and mix into the salsa. This salsa is absolutely delicious – it goes great with sliced vegetables, corn chips or even in lettuce cups. This is definitely a power packed salsa, perfect for boosting energy and antioxidant levels

- 4 ripe romaine tomatoes, chopped
- 1 avocado, diced
- ½ cup of sun-dried tomatoes, diced
- 1 small spanish onion, chopped
- 4 tablespoons of flaxseed oil
- ⅛ cup of fresh coriander
- ⅛ cup of fresh basil
- ¼ to ⅓ cup of pitted black olives
- 1 teaspoon of Celtic salt
- 1 to 2 lemons juiced
- ¼ cup of organic goji berries
- 3 pitted medjool dates

spicy miso dip ...
makes 1 bowl

1 tablespoon of miso (shiro or genmai)
1 tablespoon of red wine vinegar or brown rice vinegar
1 lime, squeezed
¼ cup of chopped onion
¼ cup of sunflower seeds
1 garlic clove
¼ cup of purified water
¼ cup of organic sesame oil
1 red chilli (or 2 teaspoons of minced red chilli)
1 tablespoon of tamari or bragg's
3 organic medjool dates, pitted

Combine all ingredients in a food processor and blend until creamy.

spinach and coriander dip ...
makes 1 bowl

2 to 3 cups of baby spinach leaves
¼ cup of parsley
1 avocado, diced
1 tomato, diced
1 lemon, juiced (plus a little rind)
¼ cup of pine nuts or sunflower seeds
¼ small onion
1 teaspoon of Celtic salt
2 pitted medjool dates (optional)
a small handful of coriander

Blend avocado, lemon juice, dates, nuts or seeds, tomato, onion, coriander, salt and parsley. Add the spinach leaves at the end with a little purified water.

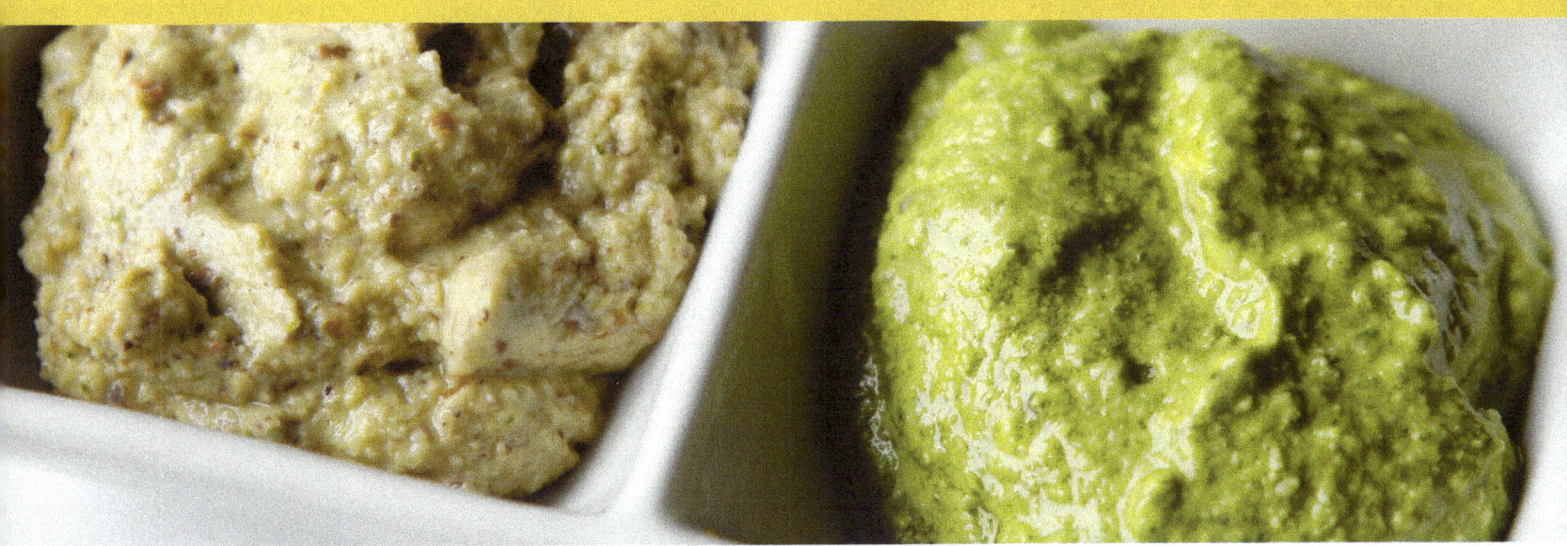

I love cheese, but cheese does not love me. Cheese made from cow's milk is high in saturated fats that clog up arteries, creates mucous and congests the lymphatic system. A high cheese intake can cause inflammatory skin conditions like dermatitis, eczema, psoriasis and acne. Eating too many yellow or aged cheeses are definitely not the best option for a healthy living foods diet. Organic goat and sheep cheeses are definitely better than dairy based cheeses, but an even healthier alternative are nut cheeses made from fresh herbs, nuts, spices and vegetables. They are high in protein, minerals, healthy fats and antioxidants. You can use these in wraps, salads, pastas or even to make healthy pizzas. Most of these last for around five days in the fridge. It is important to soak nuts for 2 to 6 hours before making these cheeses, to ensure they have a creamy texture, that is, unless you like your cheeses chunkier like cottage cheese. Always use a white nut as the base of your cheese to get a creamy, cheese like texture. From here, you can add any herb, spice or natural sweetener to create a new and magical cheese flavour.

nice 'n' cheesy ...

tex mex

2 cups of brazil nuts (pre-soak to soften)
2 lemons, juiced
2 to 3 garlic cloves
1 jalapeno pepper or red chilli pepper diced (small)
½ teaspoon of cayenne pepper
2 tablespoon of pre-soaked flaxseeds
2 tablespoons of tamari
½ cup of fresh coriander
purified water

Blend nuts, lemon juice, garlic, jalapeno, tamari, flaxseeds, coriander and cayenne with water until creamy. This is one of my favourite cheese recipes – it is very spicy, so don't make this unless you love spicy foods. The jalapeno and cayenne pepper in this cheese boosts metabolism to burn fat, improves circulation and peps up energy levels. This is a great cheese to use in lettuce or cabbage cups or taco creations

crunchy garlic parmesan

1 cup of cashews (pre-soaked to soften)
1 cup of pine nuts
2 to 3 garlic cloves
¼ cup of lemon juice
2 tablespoons of nutritional yeast, psyllium husk or lecithin granules
½ teaspoon of Celtic salt
½ teaspoon of paprika

Soak the pine nuts and cashews to soften. Blend ingredients in a food processor with enough water to make a paste like texture. Spread the mixture thinly onto teflex sheets and dehydrate at 115 F or 46 C until dry. Flip over, place on mesh screens and dehydrate on the other side until crispy. Break the cheese into small pieces and store in the fridge. I love this parmesan in my avocado Caesar salad, in soups, on eggplant pizzas or in pasta dishes

basic 'mock cheese'

2 cups of macadamia nuts, cashews, pine nut (or any other white nut)
1 lemon, juiced
1 teaspoon of Celtic salt
enough water to make creamy
¼ onion (optional)
then add ...
any seasoning or fresh herb and
sun-dried tomatoes or red pepper and
spice like jalapeno, red chilli, paprika and
something sweet like dates, yacon syrup, prunes, or other

pizza pete

1 ½ cups of macadamia nuts (pre-soaked to soften)
1 lemon juiced
¼ cup of black olives, pitted
2 garlic cloves
⅛ cup of basil leaves
½ teaspoon of Celtic salt
purified water
Blend nuts, lemon juice, olives, garlic, basil and Celtic salt until smooth, adding water until you get a creamy texture. This is a perfect cheese to serve on healthy pizza and pasta creations. Try this on the yummy raw pizza bases with tomato salsa and fresh vegetables.

macho nacho

1 cup of cashews or macadamia (pre-soaked to soften)
2 tablespoons of pre-soaked flaxseeds
2 tablespoons of lecithin granules
¼ cup of red bell pepper
1 carrot, grated
2 garlic cloves
½ lemon, juiced
1 teaspoon of Celtic salt
1 teaspoon of cayenne pepper
⅛ teaspoon of cumin
⅛ teaspoon of paprika
1 teaspoon of chilli powder
Blend all ingredients in a processor until creamy. You can add more water if you want this cheese runnier. This is my perfect nacho cheese for guacamole, dehydrated corn chips and goji berry salsa. Absolutely yummy!

salad dressings ...

The perfect way to make a salad interesting and appetising is by creating a delicious and nutritious salad dressing. I love to play around with the flavours and nutritional impact in dressings by using different unrefined oils, herbs, spices, fruits and vegetables. Salad dressings can become 'pure healing gold' if you use ingredients that pack a huge impact in the phytonutrient world. For example, if I decide to use raw apple cider vinegar in my salad dressing I am topping my body up with potassium, magnesium, calcium and malic acid to improve digestion, weight loss and immune defences. By adding into this mix a vegetable oil made from organic hemp seeds or flaxseeds I have added some amazing anti-inflammatory and heart protective ingredients. A simple addition of garden herbs can pump up the healing capacity of your salad even more. By adding 1 tablespoon of oregano I can supply more cancer protection than a whole apple and by grating in some turmeric I can provide added protection against stomach, breast, colon & skin cancer. Who would have thought that simple garden herbs that are often pushed to the side of the plate could contain so much healing potential.

create your own salad dressing masterpiece ...

3 parts unrefined oil to 1 part raw vinegar to 1 part citrus juice then add natural seasoning, fresh herbs and spices
my favourite additions are ...

juice	unrefined oils	vinegar	seasoning
lemon	sesame	brown rice	celtic salt
lime	first cold pressed olive	umeboshi plum	tamari
grapefruit	flaxseed	apple cider	miso
tangerine	hemp seed	red wine	bragg's
mandarin	walnut or	balsamic	mustard
	macadamia	coconut vnegar	
	udo's blend		

my favourite herbs to add in
basil, coriander, thyme, rosemary, marjoram, oregano, dill, sage, fennel, mint, ginger, garlic, chives, turmeric & more....
my favourite spices to add in
curry, chilli, cinnamon, cloves, cumin, paprika and cayenne
for creamier salad dressings use
nut butters, nuts, seeds, avocado, tahini, organic tofu etc

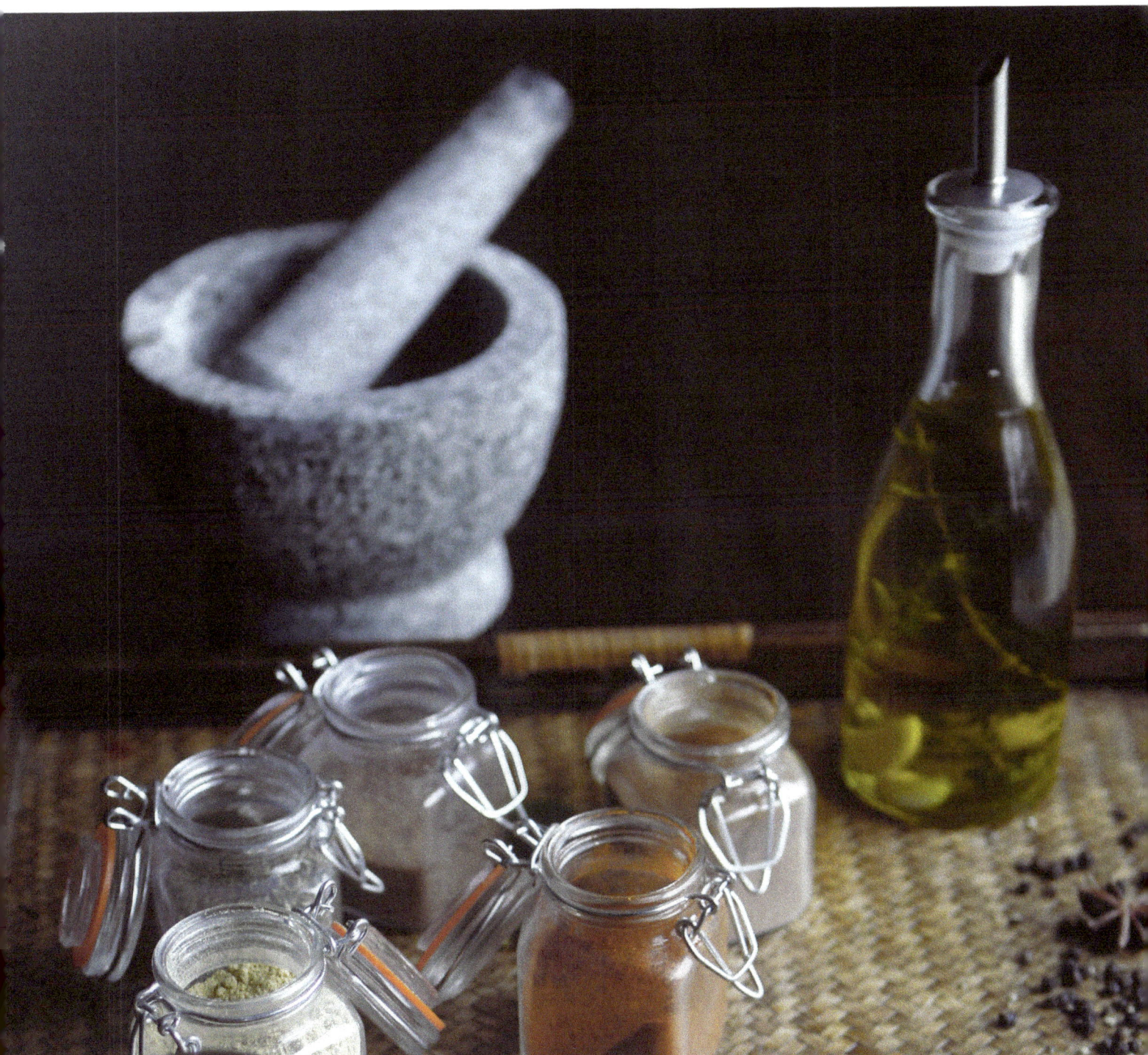

NOT ALL OILS are the SAME...

When buying oils, they should be organic, unrefined and cold pressed. They should also be found in dark bottles with no direct light exposure. Any rancidity or oxygenation will remove all of the healing ingredients found within the oil.

hemp seed oil - the KING of oils
Hemp seed oil is often coined 'The King of Oils' and it is no wonder, as it is a perfectly balanced oil rich in essential fatty acids and protein. It contains more essential fatty acids than flaxseed oil and the perfect balance of omega 3, 6 and 9 oils, including gamma linoleic acid (GLA). GLA beautifies the skin, hair and nails and reduces inflammation linked to PMS, eczema, psoriasis, arthritis, multiple sclerosis and cancer. Hemp seeds can lower the 'sticky cholesterol' that causes atherosclerosis and heart disease. This oil has a yummy, nutty taste that is perfect for salad dressings.

flax seed oil - the omega 3 superhero
Flaxseed oil goes rancid quickly - so it must be pressed at low temperatures, protected from heat, light and air, stored in the fridge and used shortly after opening. Flaxseeds are a great source of omega 3 fatty acids and lignans. These natural substances guard against menopausal symptoms and the development of breast, prostate and colon cancer. This is another heart loving oil that can reduce the risk of strokes and heart attacks. The rich omega 3 fats found in flaxseed help with lupus, arthritis, psoriasis, eczema, weight loss, PMS, fatigue and constipation.

coconut oil = the misunderstood oil
There is still a lot of controversy over whether coconut oil is a saturated fat, and therefore may be harmful to your health. Unrefined coconut oil is a saturated fat, yet it is different from most saturated fats as it is made up of almost two thirds medium chain triglycerides. These triglycerides are easily broken down by the liver and supply a quick source of energy to boost immunity. The lauric acid found in coconut oil is a natural anti-viral, anti-fungal and anti-bacterial agent that can destroy nasty microbes, fungi and parasites. Most coconut oil is refined, bleached and deodorised, a process which removes the healthy lauric acids. So when buying coconut oil look for unrefined, organic GMO free oil derived from fresh coconuts. I do not use a lot of coconut oil in my dressings, as it tends to make everything taste like 'tropical sunscreen'. I prefer the taste of coconut oil in desserts, natural ice-creams and chocolate slices.

olive oil - the heart smart oil
Olive oil is one of the best sources of monounsaturated fats. These fats help to lower the sticky 'LDL' cholesterol that causes heart disease while raising the good 'HDL' cholesterol that prevents this. It contains high amounts of Vitamin E to lower blood pressure and prevent blood clotting and plenty of polyphenols to reduce inflammation linked to diabetes, cancer and heart disease. Olive oil is also brilliant for dissolving gallstones and preventing ulcers. No wonder the Mediterranean people are so healthy!

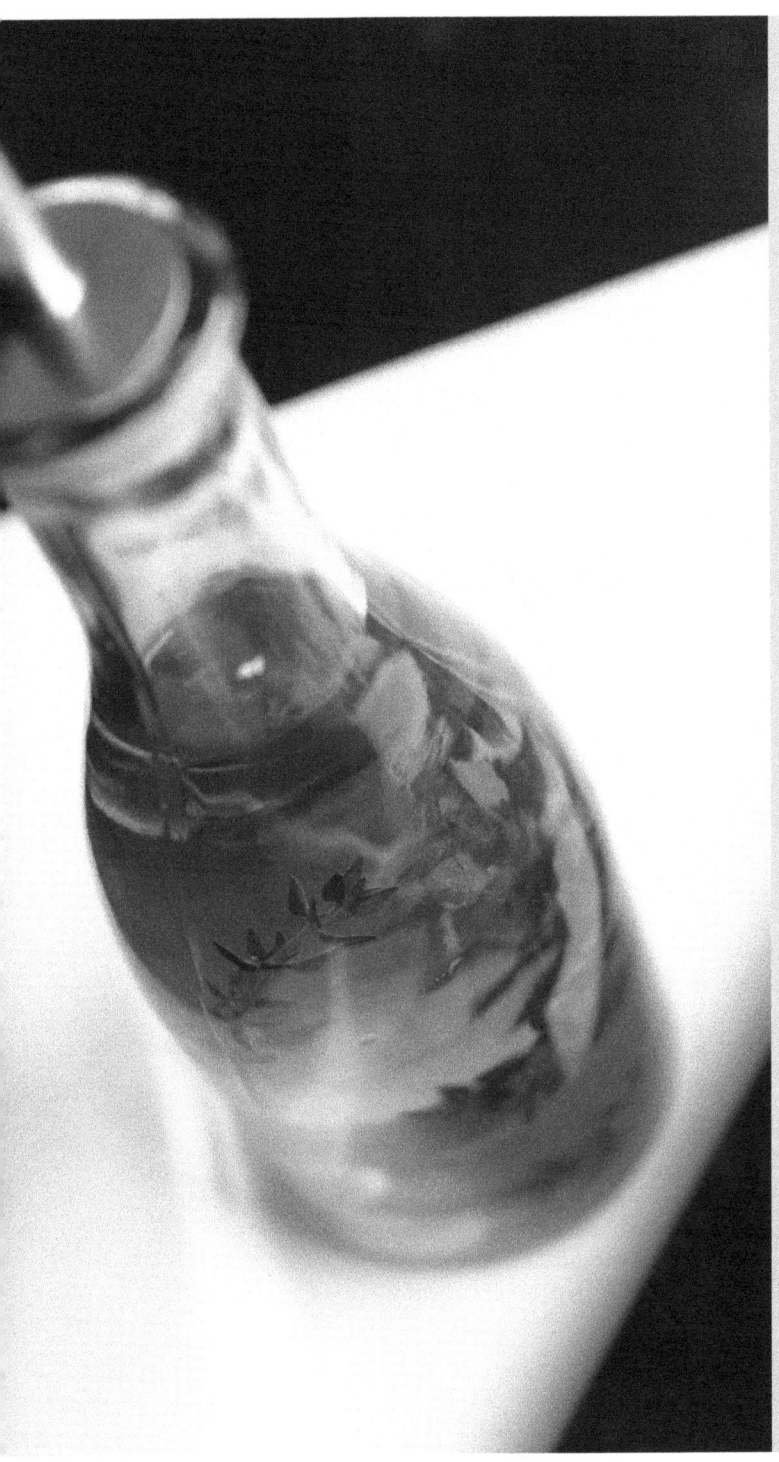

udo's oil - the beautifying oil

Udo's oil was developed by famous nutritionist Udo Erasmus. He pioneered the popularity of unrefined oils in the 1980's and wrote the revolutionary book 'Fats that Heal, Fats that Kill'. With his research into fats he created 'Udo's Oil' - a beautiful blend of omega 3, 6 and 9 oils in a perfect 2:1:1 ratio. He includes oils like flaxseed, sunflower, sesame, rice and oat germs, coconut, evening primrose oil and even lecithin. The high levels of gamma linoleic acid (GLA) found in this oil beautify the skin and hair, encourage weight loss and reduce inflammation linked to PMS, multiple sclerosis, cardiovascular disease, eczema, psoriasis, arthritis and more. This oil is perfect for improving memory, concentration and alertness. I often slip this oil into my kid's smoothies. No wonder they're so clever at outsmarting me - too much Udo's oil!

sesame oil - mystical healer of oils

Sesame seed oil has been used by Ayurvedic practitioners for over four thousand years for its medicinal properties. It contains lots of healthy polyunsaturated fats including omega 3, 6 and 9. This oil also contains lecithin to improve the health of the nerves, liver and blood vessels. Its high Vitamin E content guards against cell damage, cancer and heart problems. Ayurvedic practitioners massage sesame oil into the skin to encourage detoxification and wrinkle reduction.

walnut oil - the shy achiever

Walnut oil is a great source of omega 3 fats, vitamin B1, B2, B3, E and C, selenium, magnesium, zinc, iron and calcium. This oil can lower triglycerides and LDL cholesterol (the bad guy) while raising HDL cholesterol (the good guy). The high amounts of alpha-linolenic acid (ALA) found in walnut oil can convert into EPA and DHA giving cardiovascular and brain protective effects.

spring miso dressing
serves 4 to 8 salads

Blend all of the ingredients in a food processor. Let this sit for 10 minutes and then pour over a salad. This will keep for two to three days in the fridge

3 spring onions, diced
2 tablespoons of miso (shiro or genmai)
3 tablespoons of raw apple cider vinegar
3 tablespoons of unrefined, sesame oil
1 lemon, juiced
1 inch chunk of ginger, grated
3 to 4 pitted medjool dates

tahini treat
serves 2 to 4 salads

Blend all of the ingredients until you get a nice creamy texture. I love this dressing on any salad or even as a delicious vegetable dip. It is full of potassium, iron, calcium, magnesium, folate, Vitamin A, C, K and carotene

2 tablespoons of tahini (white or black)
1 lemon, juiced
2 tablespoons of tamari or Bragg's amino acid seasoning
1 teaspoon of Celtic salt
3 pitted small organic dates (or 2 medjool dates)
1 small red chilli (diced)
¼ teaspoon of cumin
a small handful of fresh parsley
a little purified water

siam sunrise
serves 3 to 4 salads

Blend all of the ingredients in a food processor. This dressing is similar to a Vietnamese or Thai dipping sauce. It is brilliant for boosting peripheral circulation and for lowering cholesterol levels. It is a perfect dipping sauce for the 'Thai Fish Cakes'

4 to 6 tablespoons of hemp seed oil
2 teaspoons of Bragg's amino acid seasoning
2 inch chunk of ginger, grated
2 limes, squeezed
1 tablespoon of brown rice vinegar
1 small red chilli, diced
a small handful of coriander
a small handful of parsley
3 organic, pitted dates

asian creation ...
serves 4 salads

⅓ cup of organic, unrefined sesame oil
¼ cup of wheat free tamari
2 limes, juiced
2 thai chillies
¼ cup of cashews
a handful of coriander
3 to 5 dates or 1 tablespoon of yacon syrup or 5 drops of stevia

Process ingredients, adding more lime juice if needed.
Enjoy this on an Asian inspired salad or raw noodle dish.

sweet beet dressing ...
serves 2 to 4 salad

2 to 3 tablespoons of flaxseed,
hemp seed or udo's oil
¼ cup of pine nuts
1 large beetroot, grated
2 tablespoons of raw apple cider vinegar
a pinch of black pepper
a small handful of parsley
½ lemon, juiced
½ teaspoon of celtic salt
purified water

Grate fresh beetroot and process with other ingredients. Add water to get the perfect texture. This is a delicious, sweet and tasty salad dressing that is perfect on Mediterranean or garden salads. It can also be used as a delicious dip.

beat the blues with beetroot ...
Beetroot contains betaine, a natural substance which can boost serotonin production to lift a heavy heart. If you need a good spring clean don't forget to add fresh beetroot to your juice. The beta cyanin found in beetroot cleanses the liver, lymphatics and blood stream of impurities and fatty deposits. It is a wonderful source of vitamins and minerals to stimulate the production of new blood cells while preventing infections.

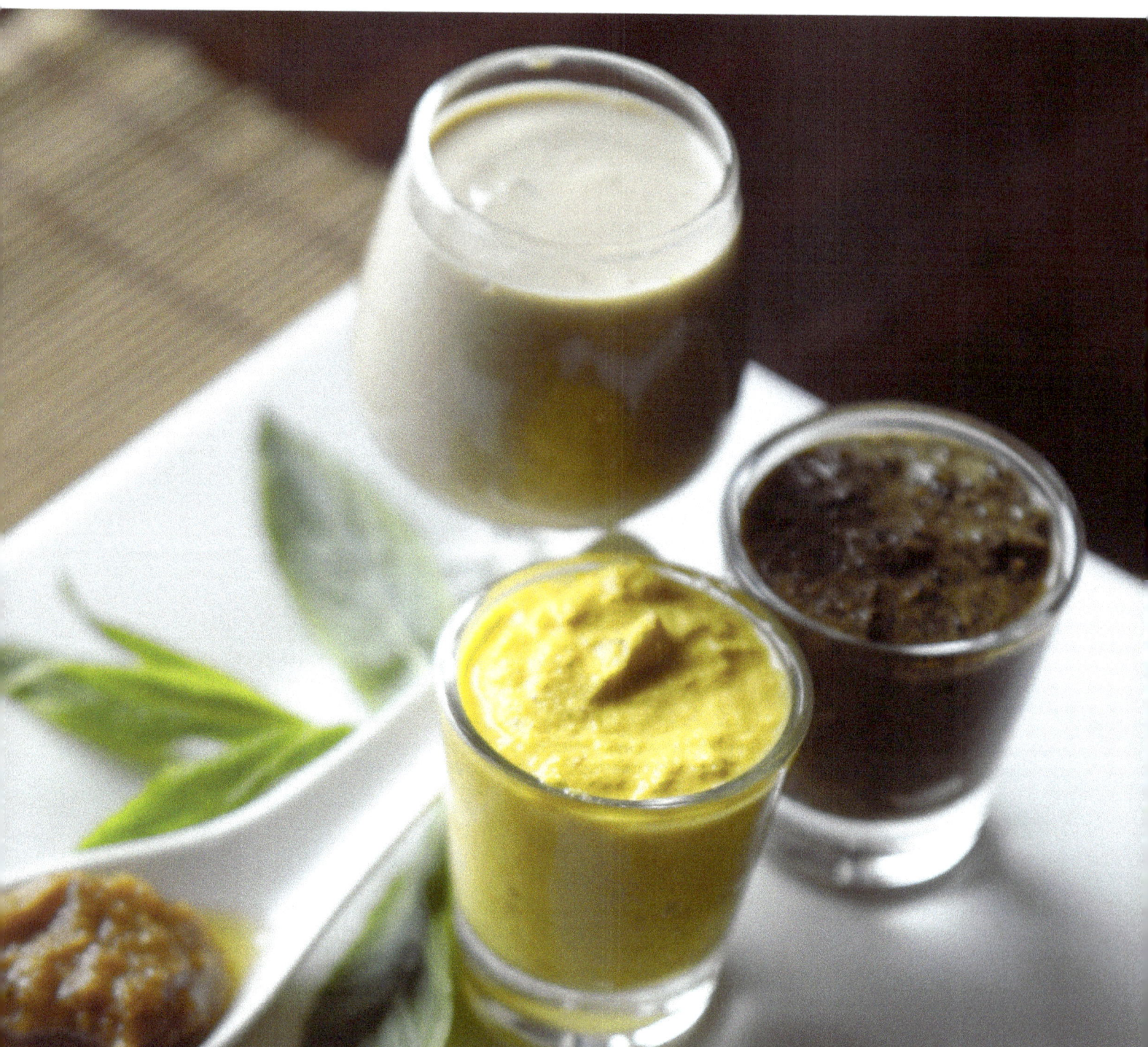

¼ cup of black sesame seeds
tahini paste
1 lemon, juiced
2 garlic cloves
2 tablespoons of miso (preferably shiro)
1 tomato
1 cup of fresh coriander
4 tablespoons of hemp seed oil

black sesame dressing ...
serves 2 to 4 salads

Process all of the ingredients and serve on fresh vegetables, salads or even use as a yummy dip.

¼ cup of cold-pressed flaxseed, hemp or Udo's oil
¼ cup of fresh lemon juice
2 tablespoons of tahini
3 garlic cloves
1 teaspoon of celtic salt
4 normal pitted dates or
2 pitted medjool dates
purified water

garlic tahini ...
serves 3 to 4 salads

Blend all of the ingredients with ½ cup of water until creamy. This is a delicious and simple satay type dressing that goes great as a vegetable dip.

¼ cup of raw apple cider vinegar
¼ cup of flaxseed oil, hemp seed or walnut oil
1 tablespoon of pure mustard paste, powder or seeds
1 to 2 cloves of garlic
½ teaspoon of Celtic salt
3 to 4 pitted medjool dates or
1 teaspoon of yacon or stevia
½ cup of almond butter

sweet mustard ...
serves 3 to 4 salads

Blend or mix in a bowl all of the ingredients. This is a very simple, yet delicious dressing that is perfect for leafy green salads.

1 red capsicum
3 tablespoons of tamari or bragg's
1 teaspoon of miso
2 limes juiced
1 small red chilli (or 1 tsp of minced red chilli)
1 small jalapeno pepper (or 1 tsp of minced jalapeno)
¼ cup of hemp seed, Udo's oil or flaxseed oil
a dash of Celtic salt

red volcano dressing ...
serves 2 to 4 salads

Blend all ingredients in a food processor or blender until completely smooth. Thin with water if needed.

hot sombrero dressing
serves 2 to 4 salads

In a blender mix oil, avocado, chilli, jalapeno, cayenne, Celtic salt, lemon juice and green capsicum. Add purified water to get the perfect texture. This can be used as a dressing or a vegetable dip to improve metabolism, cardiovascular health and energy

½ cup of organic flaxseed oil, udo's oil or hemp seed oil
½ avocado
½ green capsicum
1 small green chilli, diced
2 teaspoons of minced jalapeno
¼ teaspoon of cayenne pepper
¼ teaspoon of celtic salt
2 lemons or limes, squeezed

ginger and sesame
serves 2 to 3 salads

Blend ingredients together in a processor until creamy. This is a great dressing for green salads, Asian salads and even straight on vegetables

4 tablespoons of freshly grated ginger
2 tablespoons of brown rice vinegar
4 tablespoons of tahini
⅓ cup of sesame seeds
1 to 2 lemons squeezed
1 teaspoon of lemon rind

cool mint dressing
serves 2 to 4 salads

Process all of the ingredients, adding a little water to get the perfect texture. This dressing is fresh and icy just like a 'cool mint'. It is perfect if you are feeling nauseous or unsettled in the tummy. It is full of chlorophyll, healthy monounsaturated fats, antioxidants, calcium, magnesium and other healing nutrients to improve energy, digestion and well-being

1 cucumber, de-skinned and diced
a handful of fresh mint
a small handful of parsley
1 tablespoon of grated ginger
2 lemons, juiced
5 tablespoons of macadamia oil
½ teaspoon of Celtic salt
¼ cup of walnuts

sunny carrot dressing ...
serves 2 to 4 salads

2 carrots, grated
2 tablespoons of raw apple cider vinegar
¼ cup of sunflower seeds
¼ cup of pine nuts
¼ cup of fresh coriander or basil
2 teaspoons of miso paste (shiro or genmai)
1 lemon, juiced
a dash of Celtic salt

Blend all of the ingredients for a yummy, nutritious dressing.
If you want this dressing creamier, pre-soak your nuts and seeds before blending.

red capsicum and chilli ...
serves 3 to 4 salads

1 red capsicum
¼ cup of cherry tomatoes
a handful of parsley
a handful of fennel
1 red chilli, diced
1 lemon, juiced
1 tablespoon of raw apple cider vinegar
¼ cup of hemp seed or walnut oil
1 tablespoon of Bragg's amino acid seasoning

Blend ingredients together in a processor, adding more lemon juice if necessary.

My Calcium Soup
Creamy Tomato Soup
Red Pepper Curry Soup
Asian Noodle Soup
Tom Khai
Thai Soup
Creamy Spinach Soup
Spicy Carrot Soup
Energy Broth
Moorish Miso Soup
Sweet Corn Chowder
Sweet and Sour Shitake Soup

Delicious Nourishing Soups ...

Soups are the perfect recipe choice for obtaining huge amounts of nutrition in an easily digestible form. The texture can be altered depending on your appetite and taste – if you are hungry you can make your soup creamier with avocado, nuts and seeds or sprouted legumes. If you want a light soup, then make a watery soup full of summer vegetables like celery, cucumber and herbs. In summer, why not try eating your soup cold like a borsch and in winter, heat them up to warm up a cold tummy

my raw tip ...

In winter I am not a great fan of raw soups that are cold. So what I normally do is warm them gently on the stove, stirring constantly so I don't overheat or kill any of the enzymes in the living foods. This way I can have a warm soup that is still brimming in enzymes and antioxidants. Another idea is to place the soup in a bowl and put this bowl in a larger bowl of hot water to heat up the soup.

my calcium soup ...
serves 3 to 4

6 to 8 kale leaves
a handful of parsley
1 avocado
¼ cup of sun-dried tomatoes
¼ cup of broccoli florets
1 teaspoon of Celtic salt
1 tablespoon of pure miso paste
3 tablespoons of olive oil
¼ cup of almonds
¼ cup of sesame seeds
2 lemons, juiced
2 cloves of garlic
2 to 3 cups of purified water

Mix ingredients together in a good food processor. Add water to get the perfect texture. The vegetables nuts and seeds found within this soup are some of the highest sources of calcium in the world

creamy tomato soup ...
serves 3 to 4

4 roma tomatoes (red and ripe)
¼ cup of sun-dried tomatoes
1 small onion, diced
2 garlic cloves
¼ cup of almonds
½ teaspoon of black pepper
2 tablespoons of bragg's amino acid seasoning or tamari
½ cup of fresh basil
a handful of parsley
1 lemon, juiced
1 to 2 pitted medjool dates
2 to 3 cups of purified water

Process ingredients until smooth and creamy. Serve cold or warm up slightly on the stove.

red pepper curry soup
serves 3 to 4

2 red bell peppers (red capsicum)
1 apple, peeled
1 small avocado
½ cup of coriander or basil leaves
¼ cup of walnuts
1 small onion
2 garlic cloves
1 tablespoon of mild curry powder
1 teaspoon of Celtic salt
1 lemon juiced
a dash of cayenne
2 to 3 cups of purified water

Blend ingredients until smooth and creamy
If you want it warm, heat up on the stove gently keeping below 115 F or 46C

red is for lycopene ...

Lycopene is the antioxidant pigment that gives the brilliant red colour to certain foods like tomatoes, guava, papaya, pink grapefruit and watermelon. Research has proven its capabilities in helping to guard against several forms of cancer, including prostate, melanoma and breast cancer. It acts as a natural sunscreen and can give the skin significant protection against the sun and radiation. On top of this it can guard against macular degeneration, the oxidation of the 'bad' cholesterol and diabetes. Lycopene is an anti-ageing nutrient that beautifies the skin preventing wrinkles. Perhaps the reason why Thai women age so slowly is their high intake of papaya and guava, both rich sources of lycopene.

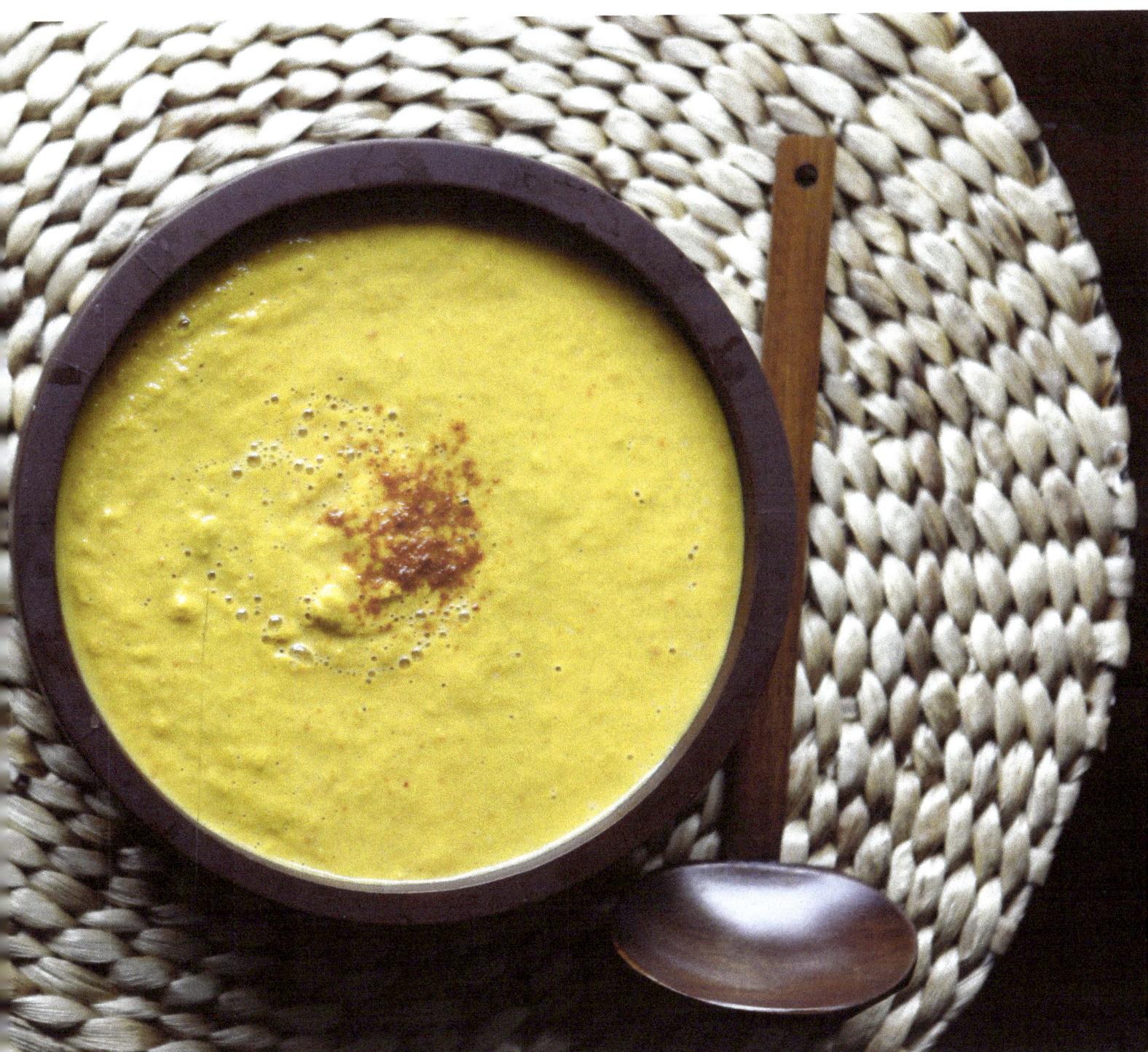

asian noodle soup
serves 4

soup base
2 cups nut milk
1 cup of purified water
1 red bell pepper or
1 capsicum
2 roma tomatoes
1 avocado
2 garlic cloves
2 tablespoons of tamari
1 tablespoon finely grated ginger
¼ cup of coriander
2 tablespoons of miso

topping
zucchini – spiralise, spirooli or shred into fine noodle strands
1 cup of bean sprouts
4 shallots, finely chopped

Blend the soup base ingredients until creamy. In four bowls, put zucchini strands, bean sprouts and shallots. If you want your soup hot, warm up slightly and pour into bowls. A beautiful Asian inspired soup

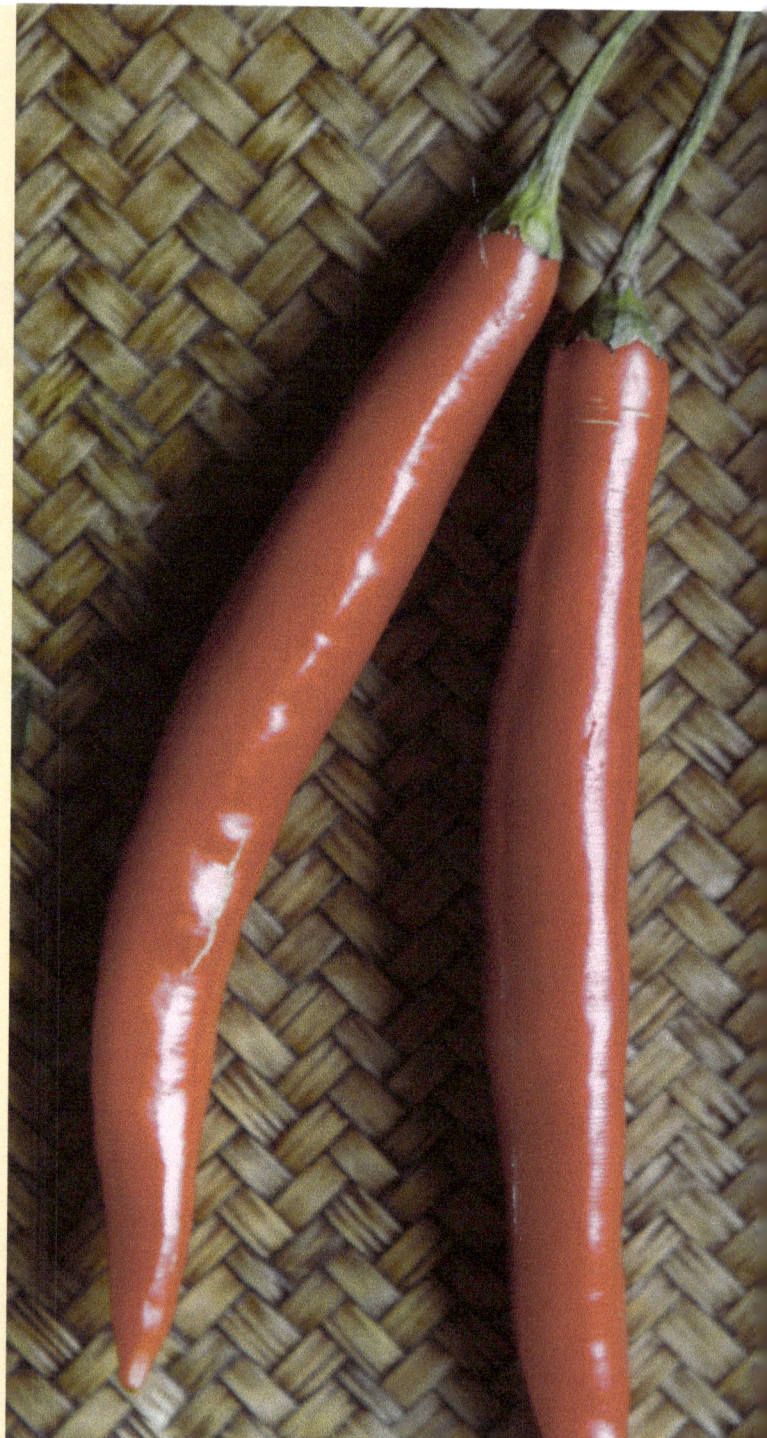

tom khai ...
serves 4

soup base
4 celery stalks
2 garlic cloves
1 inch of grated ginger
4 kaffir lime leaves
1 tablespoon of minced chilli
1 tablespoon of grated galangal
¼ cup of organic sesame oil
2 limes, juiced
2 tablespoons of almonds
1/3 cup of tamari or bragg's
1 teaspoon of Celtic salt
3 to 4 cups of water

soup toppings
10 cherry tomatoes
1/3 cup of coriander, chopped
1 cup of broccoli florets
bok choy or spinach, sliced
1 avocado, chopped
1 red chilli, diced

Blend all of the soup ingredients adding enough water to make your soup the right consistency. If you want your soup warm, simply add warm water or heat up slightly on a stove. To serve, place sliced bok choy or spinach in soup bowls. Add halved cherry tomatoes, broccoli florets, chopped coriander, cubed avocado and red chilli. Pour soup base over the top and enjoy.

thai soup ...
serves 4

soup base
2 cucumbers, peeled
¼ cup of walnuts
¼ cup of tamari or bragg's
1 teaspoon of Celtic salt
2 teaspoons of agave or
1/3 cup of pitted dates
2 tablespoons of minced ginger
2 fresh limes or lemons juiced
1 small Thai chilli or
1 teaspoon of minced chilli
3 tablespoons of brown rice vinegar
2 to 3 cups of purified water

soup toppings
1 cup of dried or
fresh shitake mushrooms
½ cup of coriander
1 red pepper, chopped
1 cup of mung bean sprouts

Blend the soup base ingredients in a processor until creamy. Warm up gently on a stove or leave cold. If you are using dried shitakes, de-stem and put into warm water to soften. Place all soup toppings into a bowl and pour the soup over the top.

creamy spinach soup
serves 3 to 4

2 cups of purified water
2 to 3 cups of spinach
(I like this made from baby spinach)
1 avocado
1 tomato
1 lemon, juiced
2 garlic cloves
4 to 6 tablespoons of tamari or Braggs amino acid seasoning
2 tablespoons of fresh mint
2 tablespoons of brown rice vinegar
1 tablespoon of olive oil
¼ cup of almonds or hazelnuts
1 teaspoon of Celtic salt
a dash of black pepper

In a food processor, blend all of the ingredients, adding water to get the right texture. If you want a sweeter soup, use fresh carrot juice instead of the purified water. Eat raw or heat up slightly on the stove

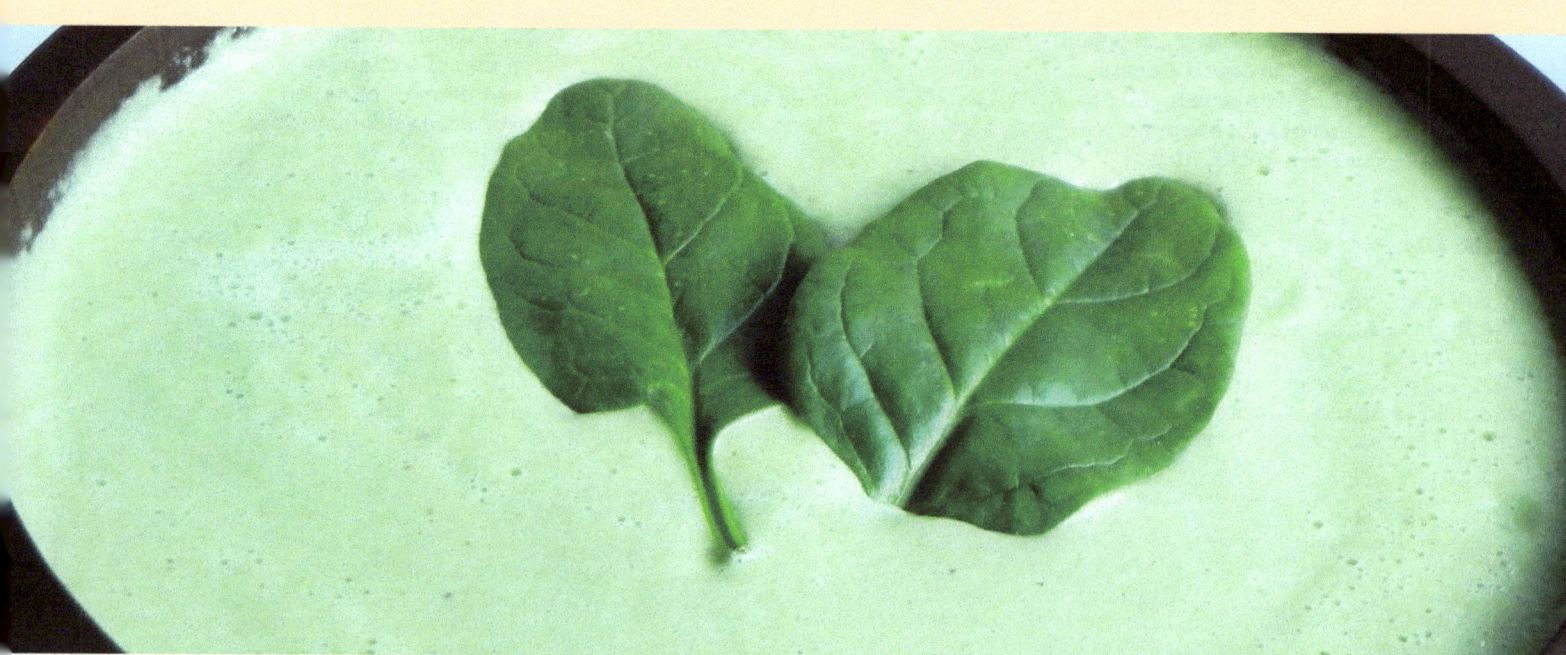

spicy carrot soup
serves 3 to 4

3 to 4 carrots
1 cup of purified water
1 avocado
1 small tomato
½ cup of coriander
1 small jalapeno, diced
1 tablespoon of grated ginger
3 tablespoons of tamari or Braggs amino acid seasoning
1 lemon, juiced
1 teaspoon of Celtic salt
3 to 5 dates, pitted or 2 medjool dates

Blend all ingredients adding more water if needed. Divide soup into bowls and put chopped shallots or chives on top. This soup is rich in beta-carotene to protect and heal the lungs, ear, nose, skin and throat and to guard against cancer and infections

energy broth
serves 3

1 cup of baby spinach leaves
1 red pepper
1 cucumber, skinned
1 stick of celery
1 tomato
2 garlic cloves
1 inch chunk of ginger
a handful of parsley or coriander
1 tablespoon of miso
½ cup of sesame seeds
4 tablespoons of Bragg's or Tamari
1 lemon, juiced
1 to 2 cups of purified water

In a food processor mix all of the ingredients, adding water to get the right consistency. Serve cold or heat up (without destroying enzymes) for a warmer soup. This soup is perfect for anyone who wishes to restore lost energy levels during a detox, after surgery or during stressful periods. It is also the perfect soup for enhancing weight loss and metabolism

miracle miso ...

Miso is a fermented soy product that can also be made from soy beans combined with barley or brown rice. A B12 synthesizing fungus known as 'aspergillus orzae' is used to ferment the grains. Fermentation can last anywhere from months to years depending on the type of miso that is used. Miso is quite high in sodium, but a little miso can go the distance providing good amounts of zinc, manganese and copper and Vitamin E, K, B12, B2 and linoleic acid. One tablespoon of miso contains 2 grams of protein per 25 calories. Its high tryptophan content ensures a good night's sleep. Miso preserves the beauty of the skin because of its rich linoleic acid content, an essential fatty acid that keeps the skin soft and pigment free. Miso is thought to offer good protection against breast, lung, prostate and colon cancer. It guards against radiation damage, helps to remove nicotine, has an alkalizing effect on the body and strengthens immunity.

different types of miso include
hatcho – made from soybeans
kome – made from rice and soybeans
mugi – made from barley and soybeans
genmai – made from brown rice and soybeans
natto – made from soybeans and ginger
shiro – made from young soybeans

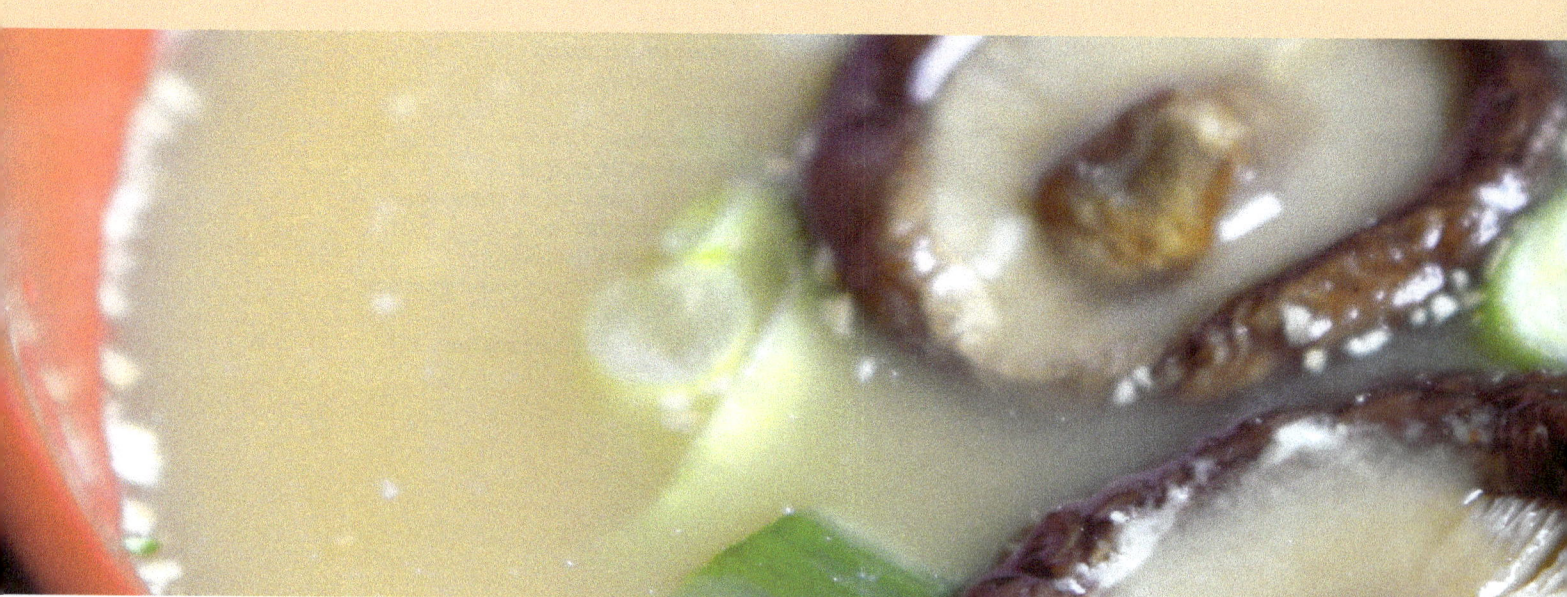

moorish miso soup ...
serves 4

soup base
3 tablespoons of shiro miso (or other type of miso)
4 cups of purified water (plus water from soaked shitake mushrooms)
¼ cup of extra virgin olive oil
1 tablespoon of grated ginger
1 tablespoon of mirin
1 tablespoon of brown rice vinegar

soup toppings
3 cups of dried or fresh shitake mushrooms
1 cup of spring onions
3 to 4 tablespoons of tamari
3 tablespoons of sesame seed oil

If you are using dried shitake mushrooms, de-stem and place in a little warm water for twenty minutes to soften. Remove and place in a bowl with chopped tofu, tamari and sesame oil to marinate. In a food processor blend miso paste, oil, ginger, warm water, mirin and rice vinegar. Add the tamari marinade to the soup. To serve, pour the soup into four bowls and add marinated mushrooms, shallots and dried seaweed.

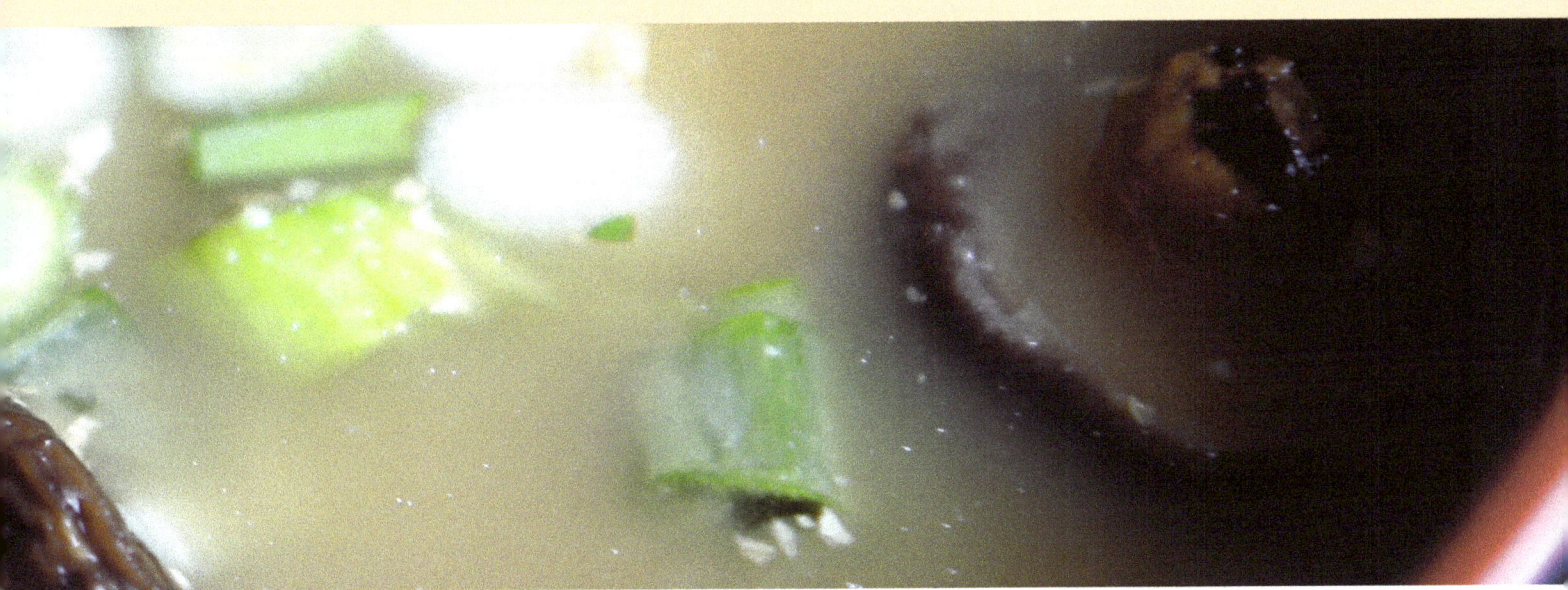

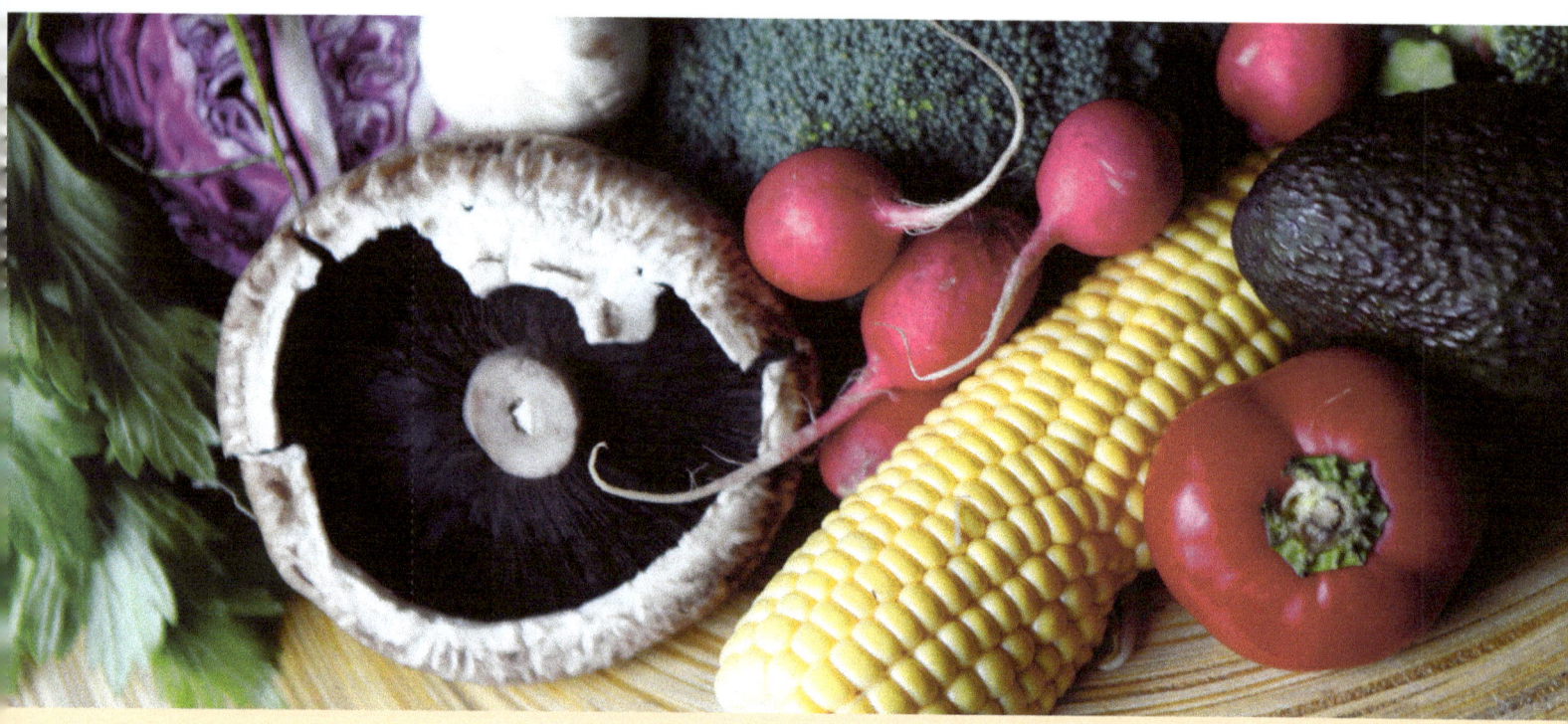

sweet corn chowder ...
serves 3 to 4

soup base
3 cups of fresh corn
1 garlic clove
¼ onion, diced
¼ cup of sun-dried tomatoes or 1 tomato
½ cup of walnuts
2 tablespoons of olive oil
1 teaspoon of Celtic salt
1 teaspoon of cumin
1 tablespoon of brown rice vinegar
2 cups of nut milk and 1 cup of purified water
(or 3 cups of purified water)

soup toppings
1 cup of corn kernels
1 red pepper, thinly sliced
1 tomato, diced
½ bunch of coriander leaves

Blend all of the soup base ingredients until nice and creamy. If you want warm, heat up gently and serve in bowls with corn, avocado, coriander, chopped tomatoes and black pepper.

sweet and sour shitake soup ...
serves 3 to 4

soup base
4 cups of purified water
2 teaspoons of galangal
2 teaspoons of minced ginger
3 kaffir lime leaves
A stick of lemongrass, finely chopped
10 cherry tomatoes
1 tablespoon of agave or 2 medjool dates
1/3 cup of tamari
2 limes, juiced
1 fresh red chilli, chopped
⅛ cup of coriander

soup toppings
2 cups of fresh or dried shitake mushrooms
(if dried, de-stem and soak in warm water until soft)
1 cup of cherry tomatoes

In a blender combine galangal, ginger, lime leaves, lemongrass, tamari, cherry tomatoes, chilli, coriander, natural sweetener and lime juice. De-stem shitake mushrooms and throw equally in the bowls with cherry tomatoes. Eat cold or warm up and pour soup mix into bowls.

Salads with Punch ...

Zesty Dill Spring Salad
Coleslaw with Creamy Peppercorn Dressing
Red Hijike Salad with a Lime Infusion
Thai Coleslaw
Cauliflower Tabouli
Japanese Vegetable Noodle Salad
Atlantic Salad
Black Sesame Shitake Salad
Simple Green Papaya Salad
Som Tum with a Twist
Watercress and Honey Soy Tofu
Turmeric Power Salad
Asian Kale Salad
Sprouted Lentil Salad
Oriental Sunrise
Baby Spinach and Avocado Caesar Salad
Chilli Infused Wakame Salad

When I choose ingredients to put into my salad, I look for different flavours, textures and colours. Vegetables are the 'key' to kick-starting the body's healing engine. They contain huge amounts of healing antioxidants, vitamins, phytonutrients and chlorophyll to help repair cells, boost energy and strengthen bones and teeth. Vegetables are also alkalising in nature. Many diseases, including cancer, flourish in acidic environments, so vegetables definitely are a disease's greatest enemy.

It is fun making a salad when you learn to experiment with the tastes, colours and healing qualities of nuts, seeds, vegetables and fruits. You can add sprouted grains or legumes to any of the salads in this section to increase their nutritional impact. Even though each recipe below has a dressing included, why not try swapping these for other dressings found throughout 'Raw Addiction' to change the flavour and healing impact of your salad. Most importantly, have fun experimenting with the ingredients in your salads and I am sure they will become your own raw food masterpieces.

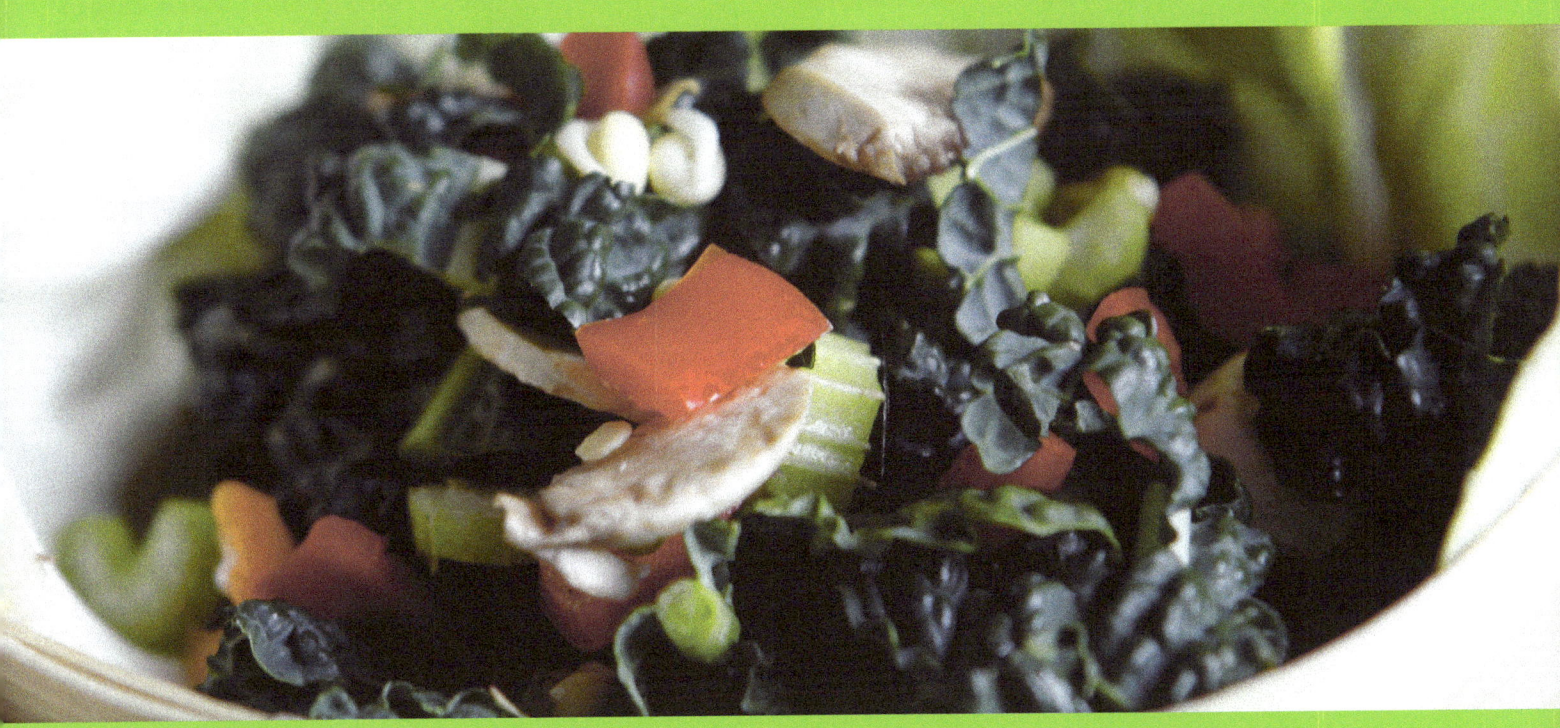

zesty dill spring salad
makes 2 bowls

salad
2 cups of kale, finely chopped
2 cups of rocket, finely chopped
2 cups of baby spinach leaves
a handful of parsley, finely chopped
1 cup of sunflower sprouts
½ cup of cherry tomatoes, halved
10 snow peas, diced
1 avocado, cubed

zesty dill dressing
6 tablespoons of flaxseed or hemp seed oil
2 tablespoons of apple cider vinegar
1 tablespoon of pure balsamic vinegar
1 garlic clove
1 teaspoon of pure mustard paste, powder or seeds
¼ cup of sunflower seeds
a handful of fresh dill

To make the salad, place chopped kale, rocket, snow peas, spinach and parsley in a bowl with cherry tomatoes and avocado. To make the dressing, process garlic, oil, sunflower seeds, dill, vinegars and mustard. Mix the dressing through the salad ingredients and let this sit for ten minutes to soften the greens

coleslaw with creamy peppercorn dressing
makes 2 to 3 bowls

salad
4 cups of green cabbage
1 carrot, shredded
1 cup of bean sprouts or snow pea sprouts
3 shallots or spring onions, finely chopped
1 red capsicum, diced
1 avocado, cubed
½ cup of cherry tomatoes, halved
¼ cup of sesame seeds

dressing
3 to 4 tablespoons of walnut, macadamia or flaxseed oil
2 garlic cloves
½ teaspoon of Celtic salt
1 lemon, juiced
2 tablespoons of green peppercorns
½ cup of cashews (pre-soaked)
purified water

Shred cabbage and place in a bowl with grated carrot, sprouts, avocado, capsicum, cherry tomatoes, shallots or spring onions and sesame seeds. To make the dressing, process garlic, Celtic salt, lemon juice, green peppercorns and cashews with a little water. Add the oil in at the end. Pour the dressing over the coleslaw mix and let this sit ten minutes before serving

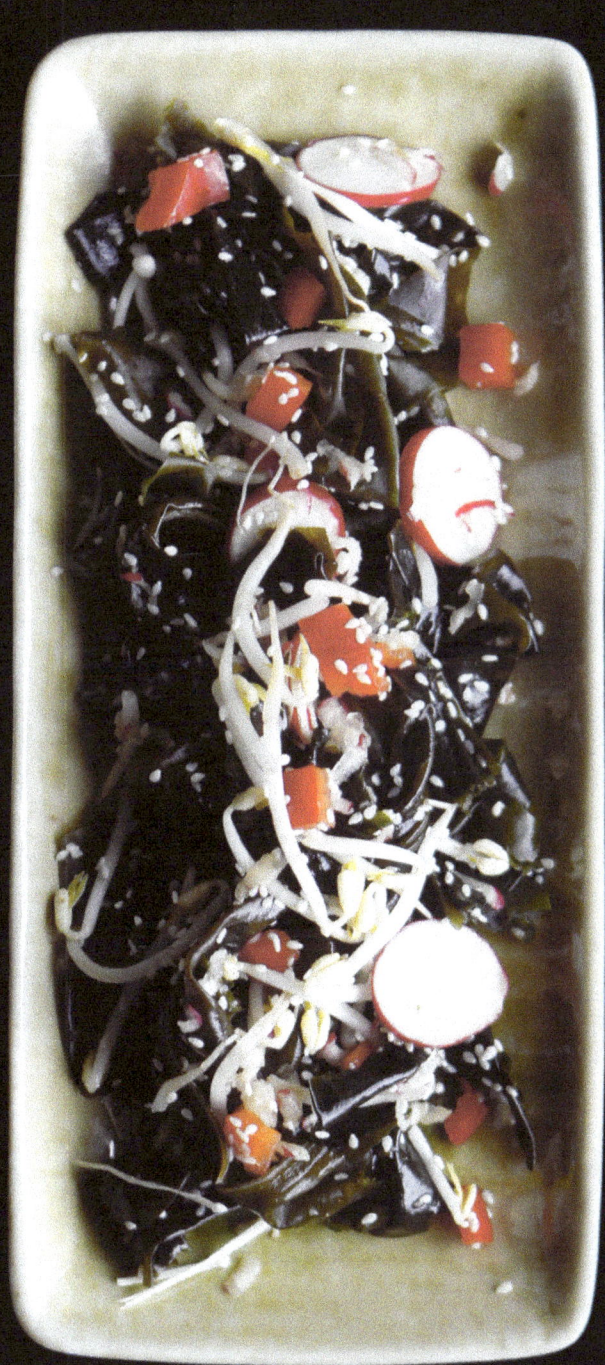

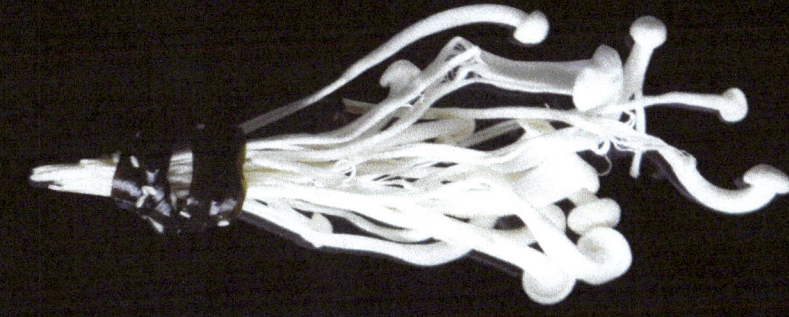

red hijike salad with a lime infusion ...
makes 1 to 2 bowls

salad
1 large bunch of kale
a handful of your favourite seaweed
(dried kombu, arame, hijike etc.)
1 tablespoon of sesame seeds
1 bunch of enoki mushrooms

dressing
1 lime, juiced
1 kaffir lime leaf
½ red pepper
4 tablespoons of organic sesame oil
2 tablespoons of miso (preferably shiro)
1 tablespoon of fresh grated ginger
a little water

To make the dressing, process lime juice, lime leaf, red pepper, sesame oil, miso, ginger and enough water to make a nice liquid. Place aside for ten minutes. Soak the seaweed in a little warm water and when soft, remove. Finely chop kale and enoki mushrooms and marinate in the dressing mix with the seaweed for twenty minutes. Place the seaweed salad on a plate and sprinkle sesame seeds on top. If you don't have enoki mushrooms, try another type of oriental mushroom. Yummy!

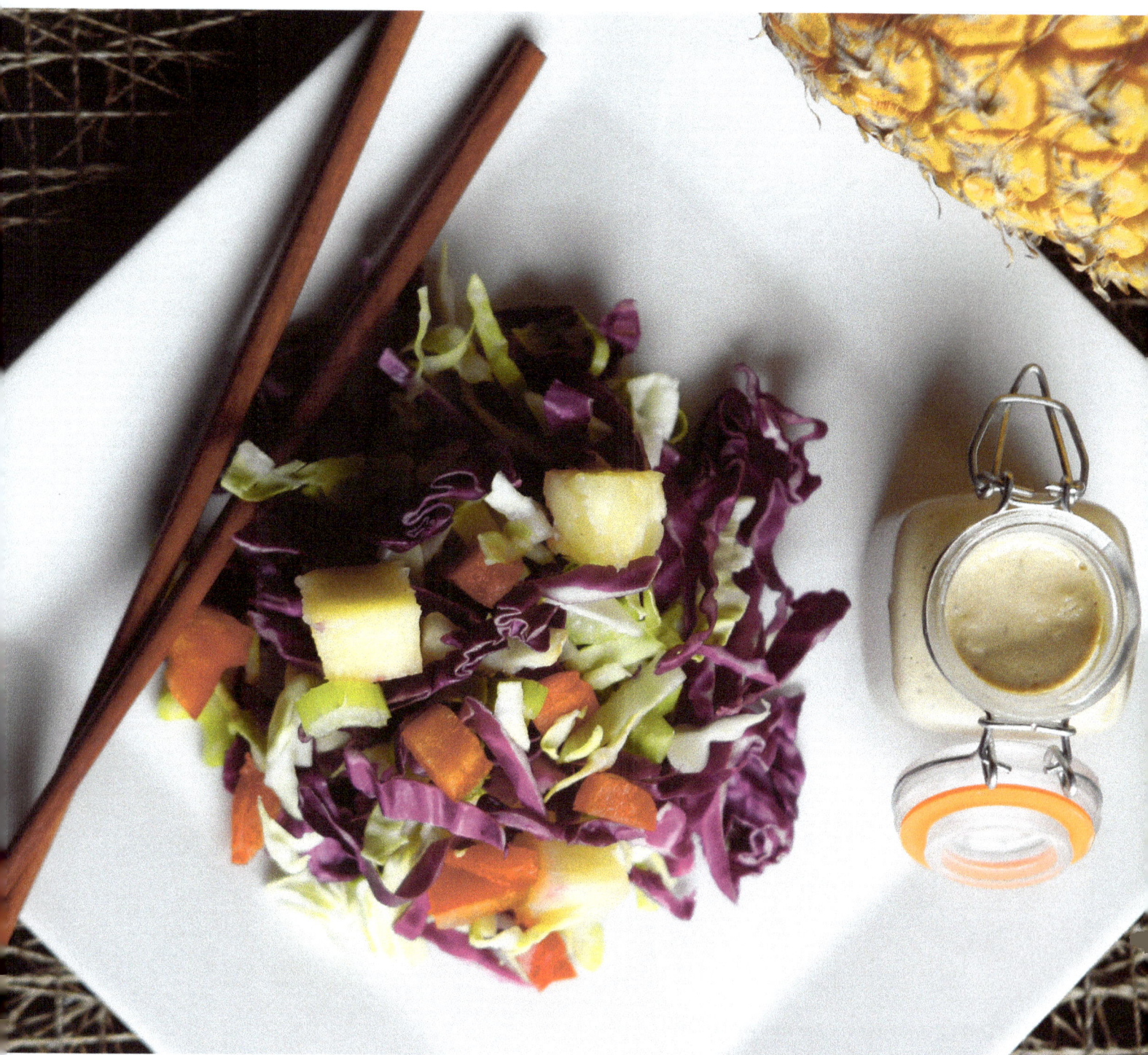

thai coleslaw ...
makes 2 to 3 bowls

salad
½ small purple cabbage, shredded
½ small green cabbage, shredded
½ fresh sweet pineapple or 1 mango, cut into squares
2 small carrots, shredded
1 red capsicum
½ avocado, cubed
2 sticks of celery
a handful of shredded coconut (optional)
¼ cup of raisins (optional)

dressing
2 limes, juiced
2 tablespoons of grated ginger
1 diced red chilli or 1 tablespoon of red chilli paste
2 tablespoons of brown rice vinegar
⅓ cup of sesame seeds
⅓ cup of fresh coriander
5 pitted dates or 2 pitted medjool dates
celtic salt

Finely shred the cabbages and place in a bowl. Grate carrots, dice red capsicum and celery and cut avocado and pineapple into squares. To make the dressing blend lime juice, ginger, chilli, vinegar, sesame seeds, coriander, Celtic salt and dates. Add water if you need to thin the dressing. Pour the dressing over the salad and sprinkle cashews or almonds through the mix. To change the flavour of this salad, replace the pineapple for mango pieces and add shredded coconut and raisins.

cauliflower tabouli
makes 2 to 3 bowls

salad
1 small cauliflower
1 cup of fresh peas
½ cup of parsley
½ cup of mint
2 spring onions or chives, finely chopped
1 avocado, diced
1 red capsicum, finely diced or cherry tomatoes

dressing
4 tablespoons of flaxseed oil
4 tablespoons of apple cider vinegar
1 lemon, juiced

Put cauliflower into a blender and pulse to make grainy. Put to the side. Blend parsley, mint and spring onions or chives in a processor and add to cauliflower mix with chopped avocado and red capsicum. Pour dressing over the entire salad. If you want extra cancer protection, add fresh or powdered turmeric to the dressing and blend. Cauliflower and turmeric when combined powerfully protects against prostate cancer. To change the flavour and healing impact of this salad, I often swap cauliflower for broccoli

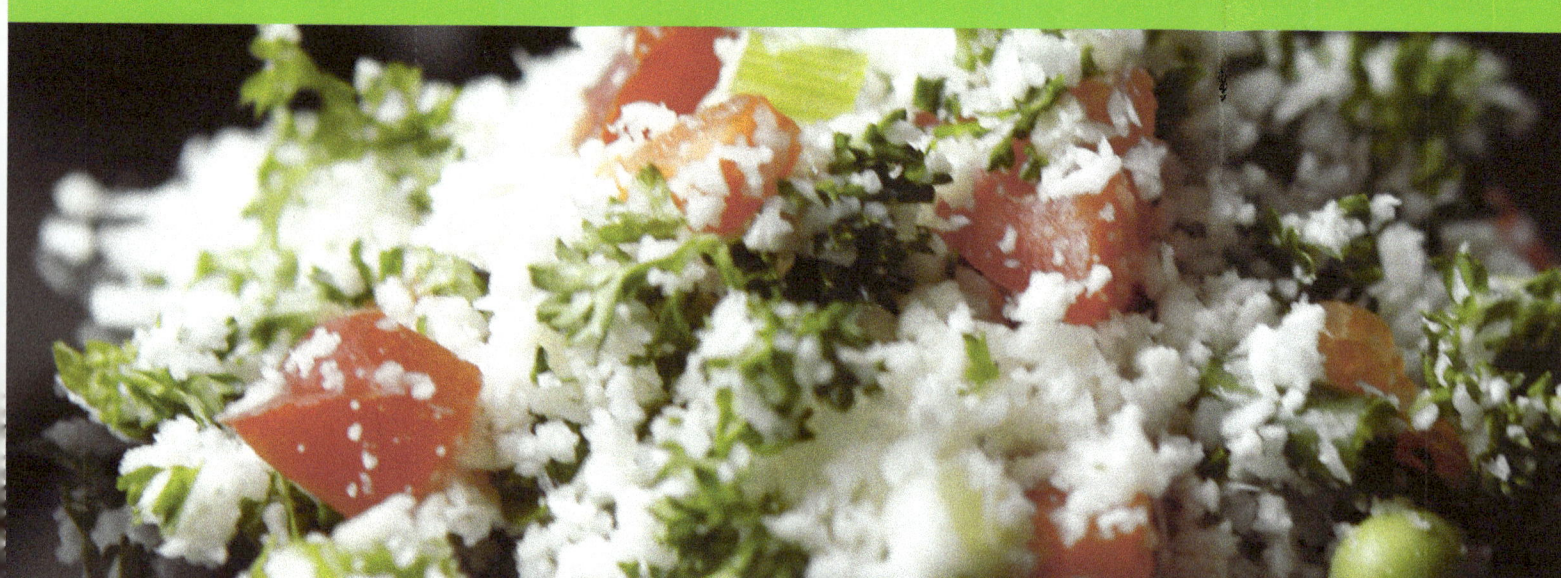

japanese vegetable noodle salad ...
makes 2 to 3 bowls

dressing
4 tablespoons of raw almond butter
4 to 5 pitted medjool dates or ¼ cup of dates
4 tablespoons of tamari
2 garlic cloves
1 tablespoon of minced or grated ginger
2 limes, juiced
2 tablespoons of brown rice vinegar
purified water to get the right texture

salad
2 zucchini
2 carrots
2 cups of broccoli florets
4 radish
1 red capsicum
1 purple onion
1 cup of shitake mushrooms
½ cup of black or white sesame seeds
a handful of baby spinach leaves
marinate - brown rice vinegar and tamari

Firstly, de-stem the shitake mushrooms and soak in hot water to soften. When soft, place in a bowl with tamari and rice vinegar to marinate for 10 minutes. Use a spiralizer or spirooli to turn the carrots and zucchini into noodles. (If you don't have one of these, simply grate the carrots and zucchini). Chop the broccoli, red capsicum and purple onion and mix with carrot and zucchini noodles. Grate radish and add to the vegetable noodle mix. To make the dressing, process all of the ingredients. Pour over vegetable mix and add torn spinach leaves and throw in black or white sesame seeds at the end.

atlantic salad ...
makes 2 bowls

salad
3 cups of seaweed of your choice
(hijiki, arame, red dulse or wakame)
3 small radishes, grated or cut into circles
1 cup of bean sprouts or mung beans
1 cucumber, diced
½ red capsicum, diced
¼ cup of sesame seeds

ginger and sesame dressing
¼ cup of tahini
1 inch chunk of ginger, chopped or grated
¼ cup of sesame seeds
1 tablespoon of brown rice vinegar
3 tablespoons of tamari
1 to 2 lemons, juiced
1 to 2 pitted medjool dates or other natural sweetener
purified water

Firstly, pre-soak seaweed in warm water to soften. Dry off slightly and place in a bowl with a little sesame oil and tamari and put aside. To make the dressing, process sesame seeds, tahini, rice vinegar, tamari, ginger, sweetener and lemon juice. Use a little water to get a nice creamy texture. Use a spiralizer or spirooli to turn cucumber into little noodles. Mix with seaweed, grated carrot and radish, diced red capsicum and bean sprouts. Pour the dressing through the salad. Let this rest for a few minutes before serving.

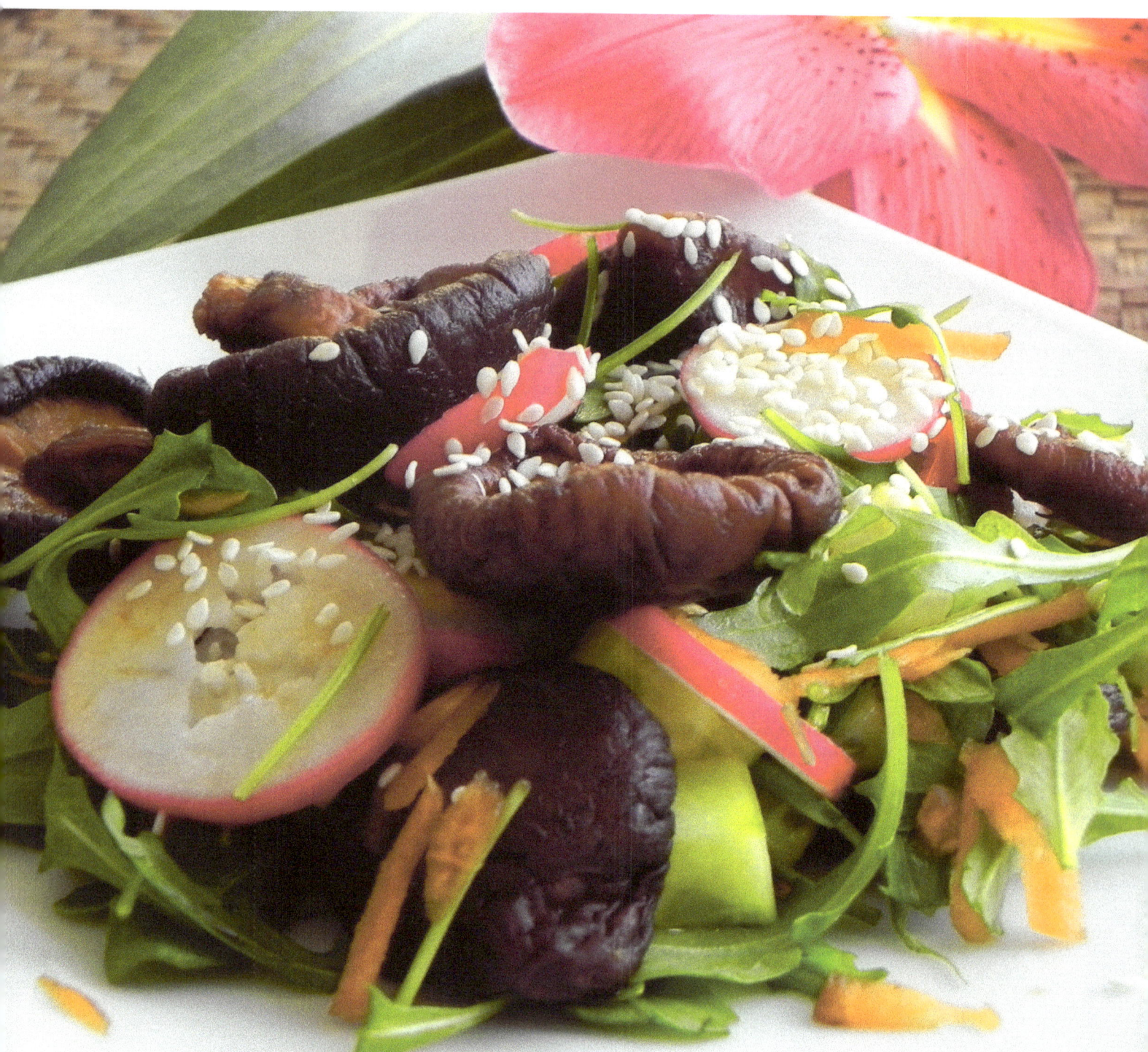

black sesame shitake salad ...
makes 2 bowls

salad
1 cup of shitake mushrooms
1 red or purple onion
1 cucumber, diced
5 small radish, cut into thin circles
1 carrot, grated
¼ cup of white or black sesame seeds
2 cups of rocket or baby spinach

dressing
¼ cup of Braggs amino acid seasoning
1 medjool date or 1 teaspoon of raw honey or yacon syrup
4 tablespoons of sesame oil
1 red pepper
2 garlic cloves
1 tablespoon of grated ginger
1 lemon, juiced

If you are using dried shitake mushrooms, de-stem and soak in hot water for 20 minutes or until soft. Remove, shred the shitakes and place in a bowl with a little tamari or braggs and lemon juice to marinate. Set aside. To make the salad, place chopped onion, cucumber, rocket or baby spinach, shredded coriander, grated carrot and radish into a bowl with sesame seeds. When the shitake mushrooms are ready, add to the salad mix. To make the dressing, simply process all of the ingredients and pour over the salad. Let this sit for 10 minutes before serving. Yummy!

the fantastic fungus ...

Shitake's are a rich source of protein, potassium, calcium, magnesium and B vitamins. They contain some powerful immune-boosting ingredients that can fight viruses and high blood pressure. Human studies have shown that only five mushrooms per day can lower cholesterol by a dramatic 12%. Shitake mushrooms have been used by Chinese practitioners to treat cancer, AIDS, diabetes, chronic fatigue, fibrocystic breast disease, gallstones, anemia, stomach ulcers and many other conditions. A powerful polysaccharide found in this miracle fungus called lentinan can activate white blood cells to defend against viruses, bacteria and stomach, prostate, cervical, colon and breast cancer. Shitake mushrooms reduce the toxic effects of chemotherapy drugs on tissues and the immune system. If you are worried about ringworm, don't forget to add a shitake to your salad to wipe out this fungus. To ensure your dried shitake mushrooms are high in healing ingredients, look for pure log-grown shitakes, not sawdust grown varieties.

simple green papaya salad
makes 2 bowls

salad
1 large green papaya (paw paw)
3 long beans (cut into 3 cm lengths) or
10 normal green beans
1 cup of bean sprouts
1 tomato, shredded
2 tablespoons of almonds, crushed

dressing
2 garlic cloves
2 to 3 Thai red chilli, diced
2 limes, juiced
1 tablespoon of apple juice concentrate or agave syrup
2 teaspoons of fish sauce (low sodium and natural)
or tamari or bragg's

Peel the green papaya, discard seeds and wash in fresh water. Finely shred the papaya either in a food processor or with a spiralizer or spirooli. If you have a mortar and pestle, pound the garlic and chilli together with green beans. If you do not have a mortar and pestle, simply use a bowl and pound with the back of a rolling pin. Blend agave or apple concentrate, lime juice, fish sauce and a little more red chilli in a bowl. Pour through the garlic and chilli mix and add papaya, bean sprouts, shredded tomato and pound a little more. Place onto a plate and sprinkle crushed almonds or organic peanuts and lime juice over the top. If you don't like hot foods, reduce the chilli in this dish. I guarantee you will fall in love with this salad

som tum with a twist
makes 2 bowls

salad
1 small green paw paw
1 small carrot, grated
1 cup of bean sprouts
1 small avocado, cubed
1 red capsicum

dressing
1 kaffir lime leaf
1 tablespoon of grated galangal
1 tablespoon of grated ginger
1 red thai chilli
2 limes, juiced
3 tablespoons of low sodium tamari or fish sauce
⅛ cup of dates, pitted or
3 tablespoons of coconut palm sugar

Peel the green papaya and finely shred in a food processor or with a spirooli or spiralizer. Place in a bowl with grated carrot, half of the bean sprouts and chopped red capsicum. To make the dressing process lime leaf, galangal, ginger, tamari or fish sauce, lime juice and natural sweetener. Add water if you need to make the dressing runnier. Pour a little through salad mix, add chopped red chilli and cubed avocado and pound with the end of a rolling pin. Sprinkle mung beans and crushed peanuts or almonds over the top of the salad mix and squeeze a little lime juice on top. A yummy European version of a Thai som tum

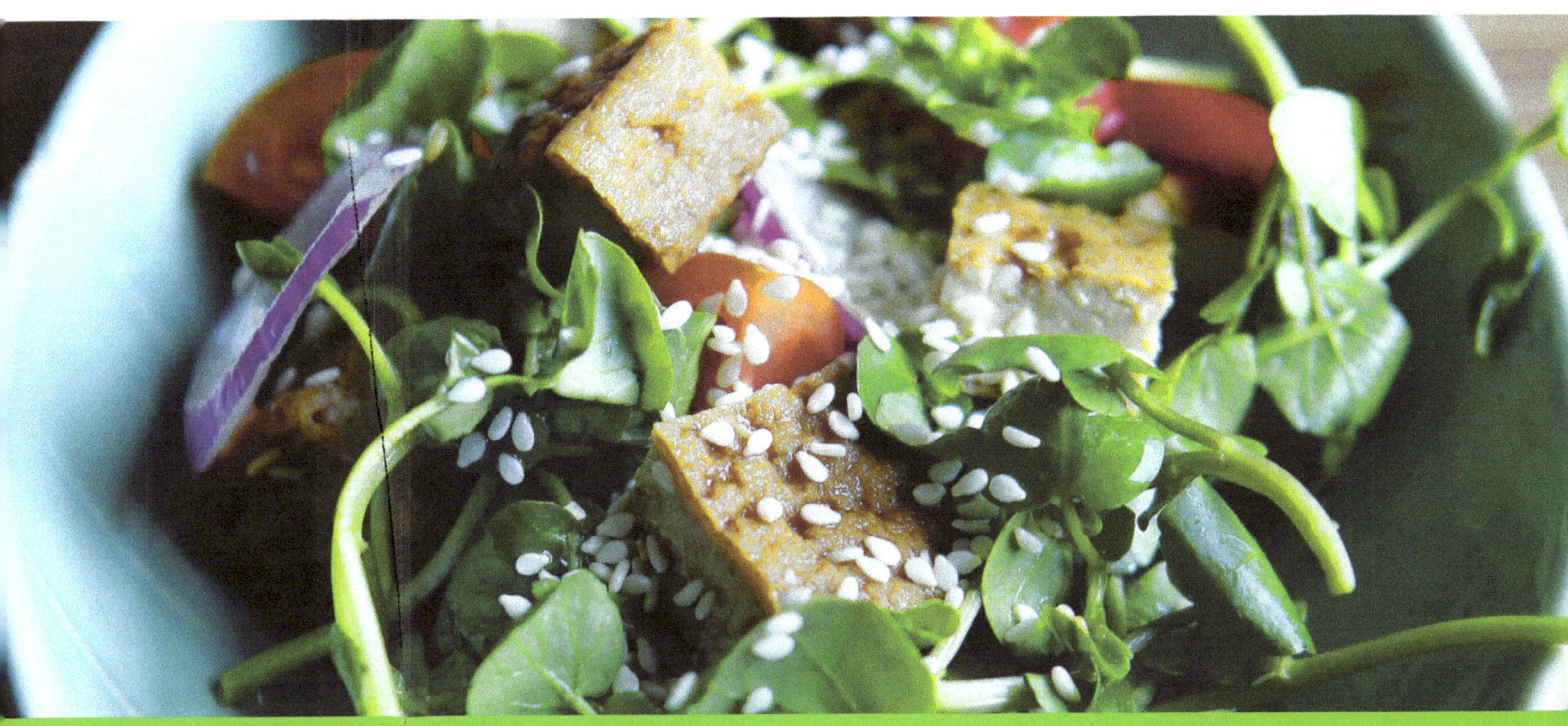

watercress and honey soy tofu salad ...
makes 2 to 3 bowls

dressing
4 to 6 tablespoons of flaxseed oil
2 tablespoons of tamari
2 tablespoons of apple cider vinegar
1 fresh lime, juiced
3 to 4 pitted dates
2 garlic cloves
a small chunk of ginger

salad
1 block of organic tofu (250 to 500 grams)
1 large bunch of watercress or rocket, chopped
1 cucumber, peeled
1 red capsicum, diced
½ cup of cherry tomatoes, halved
½ purple onion, sliced

tofu marinade
1 lemon or lime, juiced
3 tablespoons of tamari
2 tablespoons of sesame seeds
1 tablespoon of raw honey
1 tablespoon of brown rice vinegar

Put chopped watercress, diced cucumber, red capsicum, purple onion and tomatoes into a salad bowl. Cut tofu into small squares and marinate in tamari, sesame seeds, honey, lime juice and brown rice vinegar for 30 minutes. When marinated add to the rest of the salad ingredients. To make the dressing, blend oil, lime juice, dates, garlic, tamari, ginger and apple cider vinegar. Pour through the tofu and watercress mix, let this sit for a few minutes before serving. Sprinkle more sesame or sunflower seeds on at the end. If you don't eat tofu, simply leave out of the recipe.

turmeric power salad
makes 2 to 3 bowls

salad
3 cups of mixed lettuce
1 beetroot, grated
1 carrot, grated
1 zucchini, grated
¼ cup of sunflower seeds
½ cup of sun-dried tomatoes, finely chopped
a handful of basil leaves, torn

dressing
¼ cup of hemp seed or olive oil
½ cup of brazil nuts or pistachio (pre-soaked)
2 garlic cloves
1 small piece of turmeric, grated or 1 teaspoon of turmeric powder
1 teaspoon of Celtic salt
2 to 3 lemons
5 cherry tomatoes or 1 roma tomato
a dash of black pepper
a little water

In a bowl, put chopped lettuce mix, basil, grated carrot, zucchini and beetroot, sun-dried tomatoes and sunflower seeds
To make the dressing, process garlic, turmeric, nuts, oil, lemon juice, tomato, salt and enough water to make runny
Let this sit for a few minutes, then pour over salad mix

turmeric – the all round healer ...

Turmeric is one of the most powerful antioxidants and anti-inflammatory agents in the world. It reduces inflammation linked to arthritis and rheumatism and has natural pain relieving qualities. In laboratory studies turmeric stopped blood vessel growth to tumors, prevented metastasis in most tumors and guarded against breast, bladder, cervical, pancreatic, stomach and colon cancer, as well as melanoma, multiple myeloma and leukemia. Turmeric possesses anti-estrogenic effects, similar to the anti-estrogenic drug, Tamoxifen. Turmeric can improve the effectiveness of radiotherapy and chemotherapy, by reducing inflammation. It is a natural anti-depressant that encourages fat burning to enhance weight loss. It works well with inflammatory skin conditions, psoriasis, liver and gallbladder problems, poor wound healing, jaundice, Parkinson's disease, autoimmune problems and Alzheimer's. It is the rich amount of curcumin found in turmeric that is largely responsible for its powerful healing actions. To absorb curcumin from turmeric powder, it needs to be combined with olive oil and black pepper

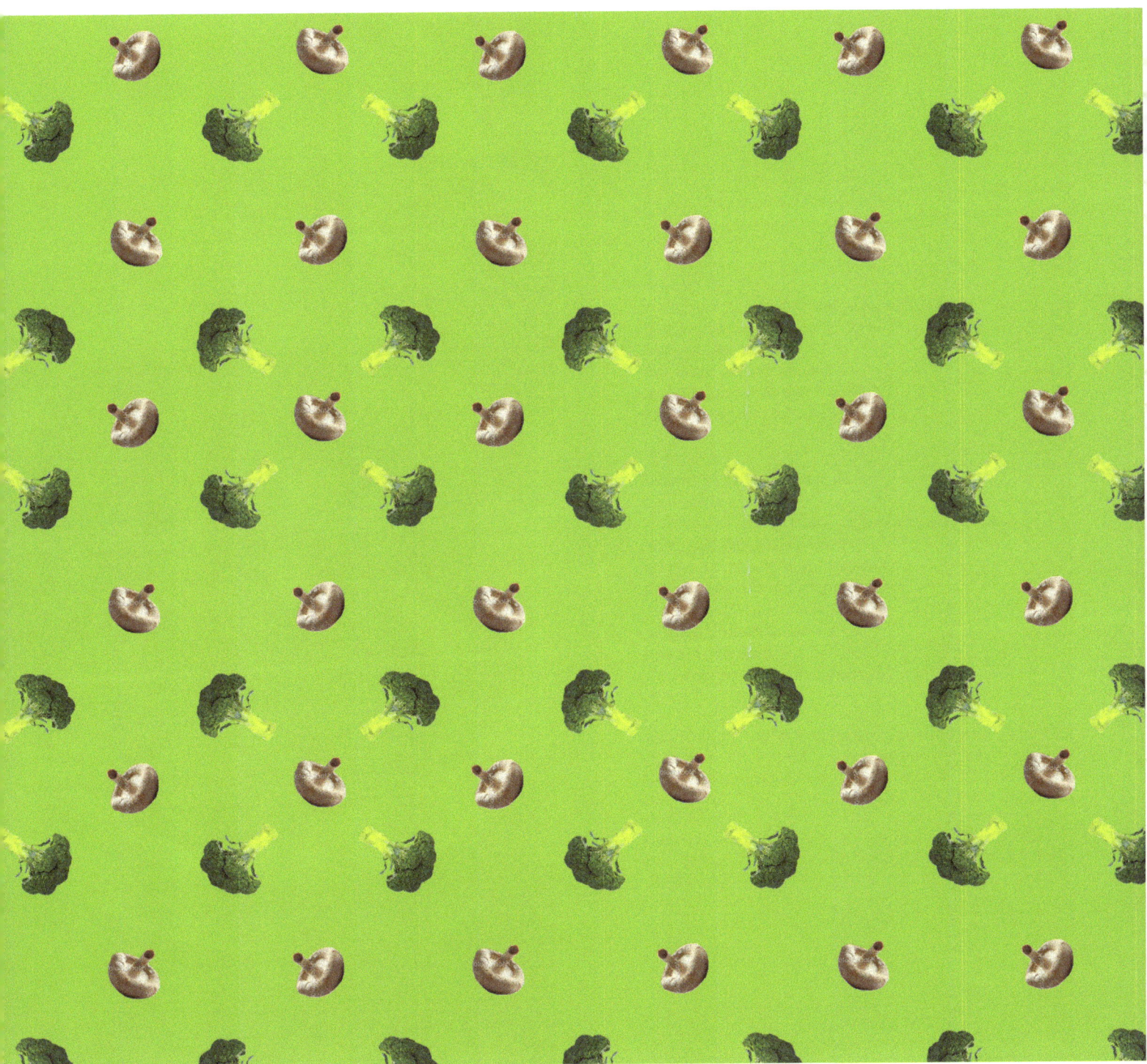

asian kale salad
makes 2 to 3 plates

salad
4 large kale leaves, finely chopped
1 red capsicum, diced
1 carrot, grated
1 celery stalk, chopped
3 to 4 mushrooms, sliced
a handful of bean sprouts

dressing
6 tablespoons of tahini
1 kaffir lime leaf
2 teaspoons of bragg's amino acid seasoning
2 pitted medjool dates or
1 tablespoon of yacon or agave
½ cup of coriander leaves
¼ cup of purified water
1 teaspoon of grated ginger
2 garlic cloves
4 tablespoons of sesame seed oil

Finely chop kale and place in a bowl with a little bragg's and lemon juice. Marinate for ten minutes. To make the dressing, process tahini, braggs, lime leaf, dates, coriander, ginger, garlic, oil and water. Set aside for 10 minutes. Add carrot, red capsicum, celery, mushrooms and sprouts to the kale mix. Pour dressing over the top and sprinkle with pumpkin seeds. Delicious!

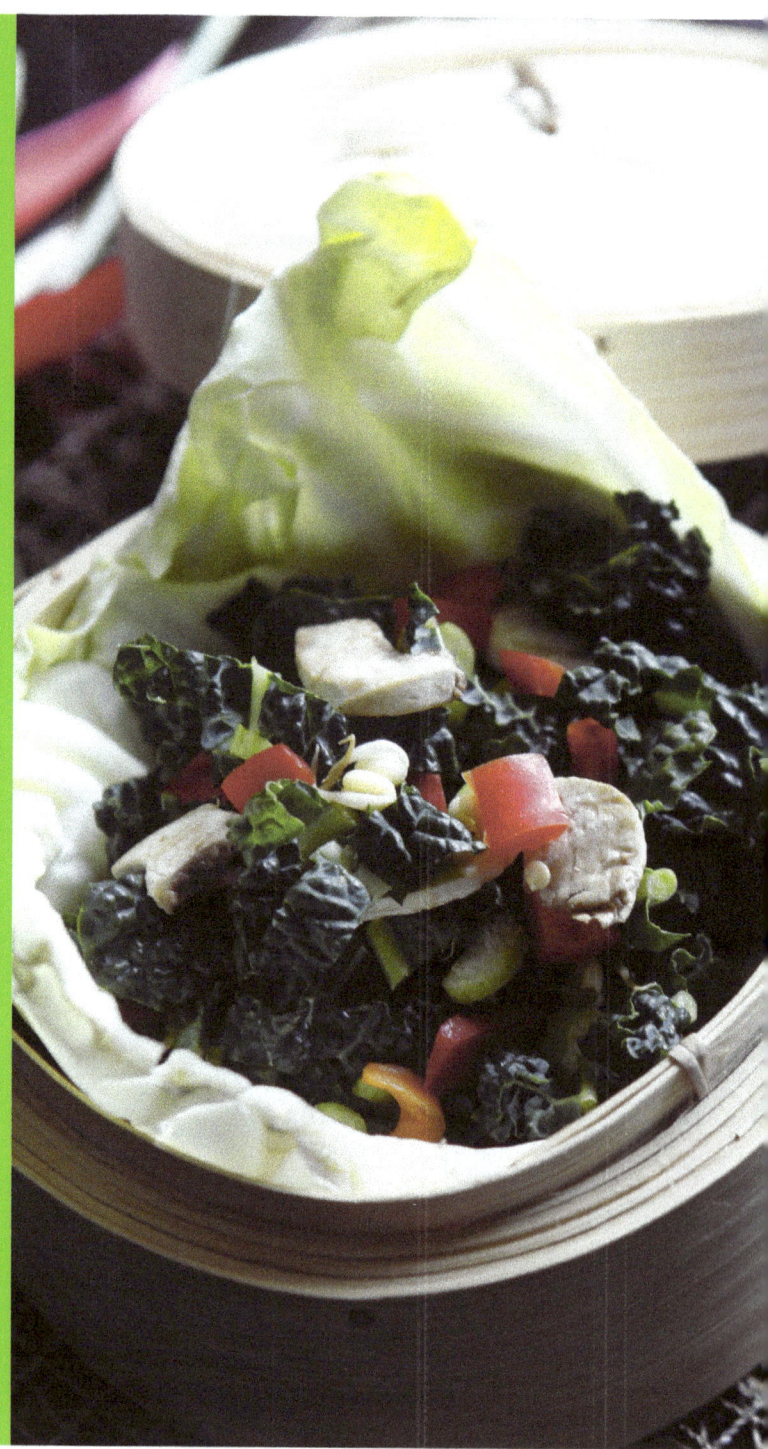

sprouted lentil salad ...
makes 2 to 3 bowls

salad
- 2 cups of sprouted lentils
- ½ cup of cherry tomatoes, quartered
- ½ purple onion, chopped
- 1 red capsicum, finely chopped
- a handful of parsley, finely chopped

coriander and lime dressing
- 4 tablespoons of flaxseed, Udo's or olive oil
- 2 limes, juiced
- 3 tablespoons of apple cider vinegar
- ½ teaspoon of Celtic salt
- 1 cup of coriander

To make the dressing, blend coriander, oil, lime juice, apple cider vinegar and Celtic salt. In a separate mixing bowl, combine the lentils, onion, capsicum, tomatoes and parsley. Pour the dressing through the salad mix and leave for five minutes before serving.

oriental sunrise ...
makes 2 bowls

salad
- 1 cup of spinach leaves
- 2 cups of bok choy or tat soi or mizuna
- 1 cup of rocket, torn into pieces
- a handful of coriander
- 1 cup of cherry tomatoes, halved
- 1 red capsicum, diced
- 1 carrot, grated

dressing
- 1 avocado
- 4 tablespoons of flaxseed oil
- 2 tablespoons of tamari
- 1 teaspoon of minced or grated ginger
- 2 tablespoons of almond or hazelnut butter
- 2 tablespoons of sesame seeds
- 2 tablespoons of apple cider vinegar
- 1 to 2 limes, juiced

To make the salad, chop Asian salad greens and add to torn rocket and baby spinach leaves. Put into a bowl with shredded coriander, cherry tomatoes, red capsicum and grated carrot. To make the dressing, process avocado, oil, tamari, ginger, nut butter, sesame seeds, apple cider vinegar and lime juice. Toss through the salad mix and let this sit for ten minutes before serving. For added flavour, sprinkle chopped almonds through the salad.

baby spinach and avocado caesar salad
makes 3 bowls

salad
4 cups of baby spinach leaves
2 cups of mixed lettuce
1 cup of black olives (naturally ripened)
1 avocado
½ cup of cherry tomatoes, halved
¼ cup of walnuts
¼ cup of garlic parmesan
(see recipe in 'condiments, spreads and dips')

dressing
½ cup of cashews (pre-soaked)
1 lemon, juiced
1 roma tomato
1 teaspoon of mustard paste, powder or seeds
4 to 6 tablespoons of flaxseed or walnut oil
2 garlic cloves
a handful of parsley
1 teaspoon of celtic salt

In a bowl place spinach and lettuce with chopped olives, avocado and cherry tomatoes. To make the dressing, process lemon juice, cashews, mustard, oil, garlic, parsley, tomato and salt. Pour over the salad mix and sprinkle walnuts and garlic parmesan through. This is a healthier version of traditional Caesar salad. The simple mayo dressing also goes perfectly with this salad

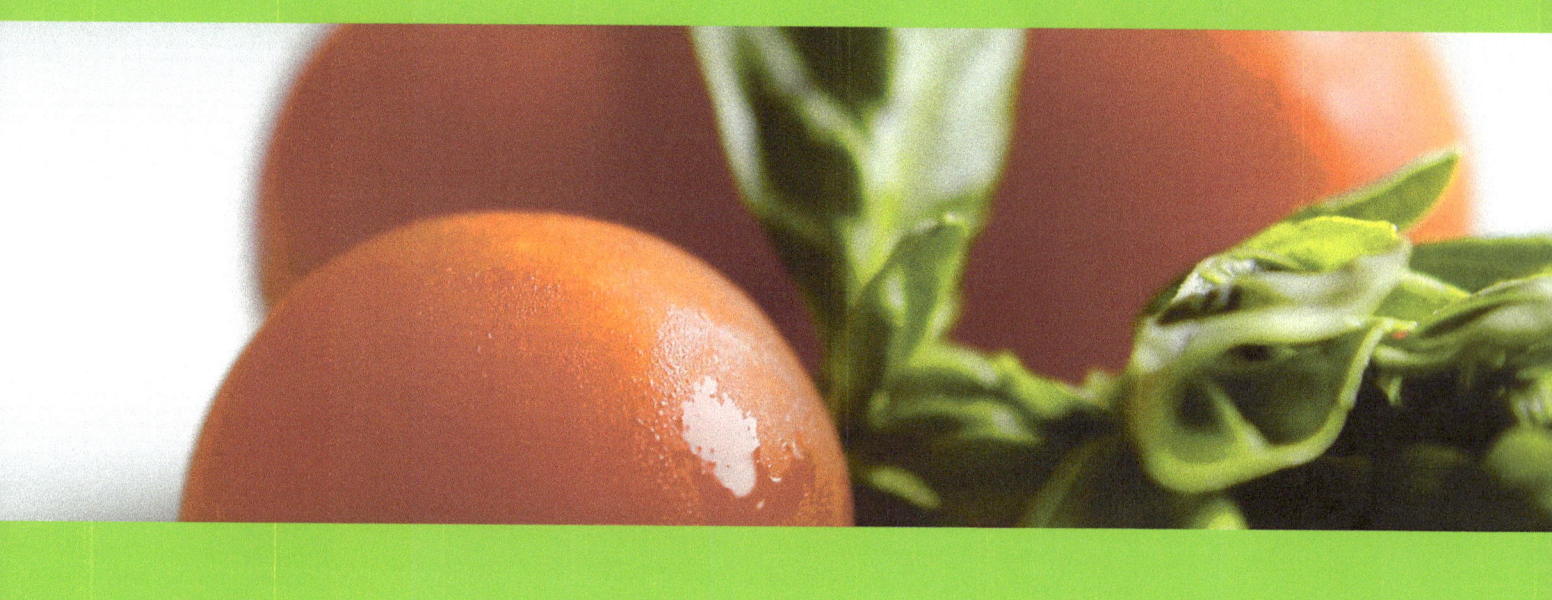

chilli infused wakame salad ...
makes 2 bowls

salad
3 cups of dried wakame
1 cup of bean sprouts
1 carrot
2 spring onions

marinade
3 tablespoons of tamari
1 red chilli, finely chopped
1 lime, juiced

dressing
2 tablespoons of tamari
2 tablespoons of brown rice vinegar
3 tablespoons of hemp seed or sesame oil
1 pitted medjool date or
1 teaspoon of agave, yacon or raw honey
1 tablespoon of miso (preferably shiro)
1 garlic clove
1 fresh lemon, juiced
water to dilute

Soak the wakame in water for a few minutes or until soft.
Drain and then marinate in tamari, lime juice and chopped red chilli.
To make the dressing, blend tamari, rice vinegar, natural sweetener, oil, miso, garlic, lemon juice and water if needed.
Put wakame, bean sprouts, carrot and chopped spring onions into a bowl.
Pour the dressing over the top and sprinkle toasted sesame seeds through the mix.

Pasta with Passion
Fake Spaghetti Bolognaise
Pad Thai
Vegetable Gado Gado
Chilli and Red Pepper Linguine

Guilt Free Burgers
Spicy Turmeric Tofu Fillets
Sun Burgers
Curried Nut Burgers
Raw Thai Fish Cakes

Burrito Cups
Southern Burrito Cups
Mediterranean Burrito Cups
Oriental Burrito Cups

Mock Sushi
Rice-free Sushi Rolls
Cauliflower Sushi
Pickled Ginger

Curry in a Hurry
Thai Red Curry with Noodles
Tibetan Antioxidant Curry
Sprouted Dhal

More Mains to Die For
Peppered Garlic Tofu
Creamy Olive Dip in Vegetable Cups
Stuffed Bell Pepper Mushrooms
Mediterranean Tomato Cups
Eggplant Pizzas
Vietnamese Cabbage Rolls with Dipping Sauce

Mains to die for ...

Traditional 'Italian' pasta dishes made the old fashioned way were healthy as they contained simple, healing ingredients like tomatoes, garlic, olive oil and basil. Their pasta was also made from unprocessed grains that were not stored for long periods of time. Modern and westernized pasta dishes are completely different. They are made from highly processed glutinous pasta dripping in sugar rich sauces. One cup of refined wheat pasta converts to 43 grams of carbohydrates or 36 grams of starch or sugar. That is around seven teaspoons of sugar in one cup of pasta.

A healthy version of pasta can be made from lots of different vegetables. By using a spiralizer or a spirooli you can create beautiful, long strands of pasta from squash, zucchini, beetroot or other types of vegetables. Simply make a yummy healthy pesto, marinara or alfredo sauce with a similar texture to normal pasta sauces, but without the unwanted carbohydrates, starch, gluten and sugar.

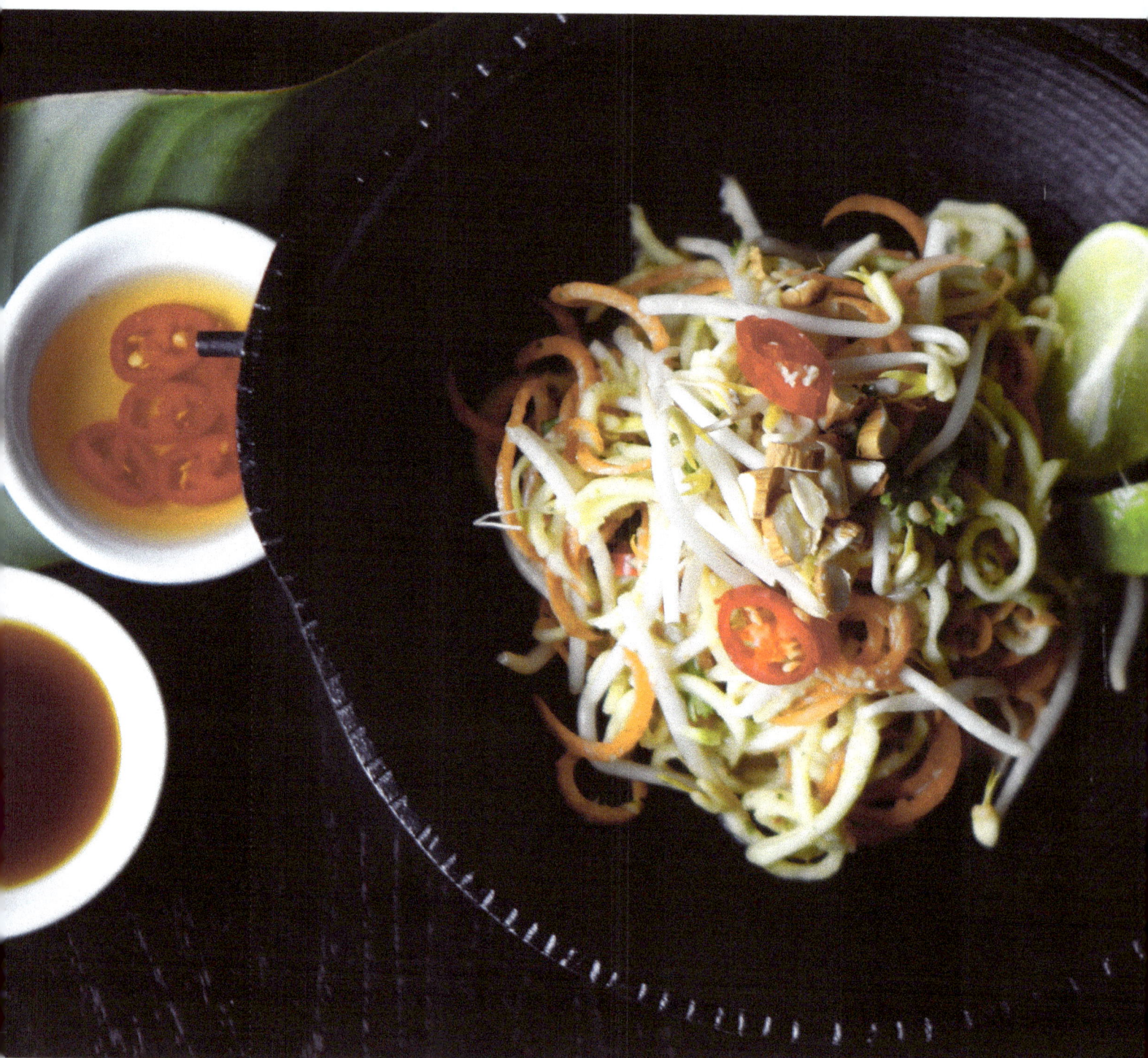

pad thai...

makes 4 serves

Pad Thai is definitely one of my favourite Thai dishes. Unfortunately traditional Pad Thai is made with lots of sugar, fish sauce and vegetable oil. So rather than giving up on this beautiful exotic dish, I now make a healthy, yummy version of Pad Thai.

noodles

1 yellow or white onion, marinated
4 zucchini
2 carrots
1 tomato, shredded
1 cup of bean sprouts
a handful of coriander

marinade

4 tablespoons of tamari or Bragg's
4 tablespoons of brown rice vinegar

sauce

1 teaspoon of grated galangal
2 limes, juiced
5 to 6 organic, pitted dates or 3 pitted medjool dates
2 tablespoons of Bragg's or
1 tbsp of pure fish sauce – made from anchovies or sardines
1 tablespoon of brown rice vinegar
2 to 3 kaffir lime leaves
½ cup of pure almond butter
¼ to ½ cup of purified water
½ cup of coriander
2 thai red chillies (optional)

To make the noodles, marinate sliced onion in a little tamari and rice vinegar for around 10 minutes. Spirooli or spiralize carrots and zucchini. Cut red capsicum into slices and combine all of the ingredients in a bowl with sprouts and marinated onion. Finely chop up one red chilli and add to the noodle bowl with lime juice and coriander. Set aside.

To make the sauce blend galangal, one red chilli, lime juice, dates, coriander, braggs or fish sauce, rice vinegar, almond butter, kaffir lime leaves and a little water and blend until smooth. Toss noodles with sauce before serving. Let this sit for a few minutes, then place on four plates with sprouts, crushed almonds or organic peanuts and torn coriander. Sprinkle a little lime juice over the top of each. Absolutely delicious and very authentic!

noodles
4 summer zucchini
2 yellow squash
1 serve of 'nutty meat' (optional)

sauce
3 to 4 tomatoes
1 cup of sun-dried tomatoes
2 to 3 garlic cloves
(depending on how spicy you want it)
½ bunch of fresh basil
2 tablespoons of fresh oregano
½ white or yellow onion
¼ cup of cold pressed olive oil
¼ cup of lemon juice
½ cup of pitted dates
1 teaspoon of Celtic salt
1 tablespoon of tamari

fake spaghetti bolognaise ...
makes 3 serves

To make the pasta, cut off the top and bottom of the zucchini and squash and place in the spiralizer or spirooli to make long spaghetti noodles. Place pasta into a bowl with olive oil and celtic salt and set aside.

To make the sauce process tomatoes, garlic, basil, oregano, onion, lemon juice, dates, celtic salt, oil and tamari until creamy. If you want your sauce runnier, add more water. To get a meatier type bolognaise, stir nutty meat through the pasta sauce or form the nutty meat into balls and dehydrate to make 'fake meatballs'. Place a little baby spinach and black olives on 3 to 4 plates and pour the sauce over the top. Squeeze with lemon juice and add a little garlic parmesan for extra flavour.

noodles
2 zucchini
2 summer squash
1 beetroot
½ cup of black olives, diced
½ cup of sun-dried tomatoes or cherry tomatoes

sauce
2 red capsicum
1 lemon squeezed
1 garlic clove
2 tablespoons of flaxseed or macadamia oil
1 teaspoon of Celtic salt
1 cup of cashews or pine nuts
¼ cup of basil leaves
1 to 2 teaspoons of red chilli paste

chilli and red pepper linguine ...
makes 3 serves

To make the noodles, use a spirooli to create long pasta strands from zucchini, squash and beetroot. Divide evenly between four bowls. Throw black olives and sun-dried tomatoes into each bowl with a handful of pine nuts.

To make the sauce, process capsicum, lemon juice, garlic, oil, celtic salt, pine nuts, basil and chilli paste until creamy. Pour sauce over pasta and top with crunchy home-made parmesan.

vegetable gado gado ...
makes 4 serves

vegetable mix
2 carrots
1 red capsicum
1 cup of bean sprouts
2 cups of green cabbage
1 purple onion
10 green beans
2 celery stalks
½ cup of cashews, almonds or peanuts
a handful of coriander

gado gado sauce 1 (spicy version)
2 teaspoons of grated or minced ginger
2 limes, juiced
2 to 3 pitted medjool dates
2 tablespoons of tamari
1 tablespoon of brown rice vinegar
1 cup of pure almond butter (or crushed peanuts for a traditional sauce)
¼ cup of purified water
2 garlic cloves
2 small bird chillies (if you like it hot, like me)

gado gado sauce 2 (not spicy)
3 tablespoons of almond butter
1 lemon, juiced
2 tablespoons of tamari
2 tablespoons of sesame oil
2 to 3 pitted medjool dates
¼ teaspoon of celtic salt
purified water

Spirooli or spiralize the zucchini and carrot (or grate). Slice up red capsicum, cut green beans into 2 inch lengths, dice purple onion, shred cabbage and dice celery. Put into a bowl with bean sprouts. Finely chop up red chillies and add to the vegetable mix with torn coriander. To make either gado gado sauce, simply process all of the ingredients together adding water if necessary. If you have no problem with peanuts, use organic peanuts instead of almond butter for a more authentic sauce. Toss vegetables with sauce before serving. Place onto four plates and top with bean sprouts, crushed nuts and torn coriander.

guilt free burgers ...

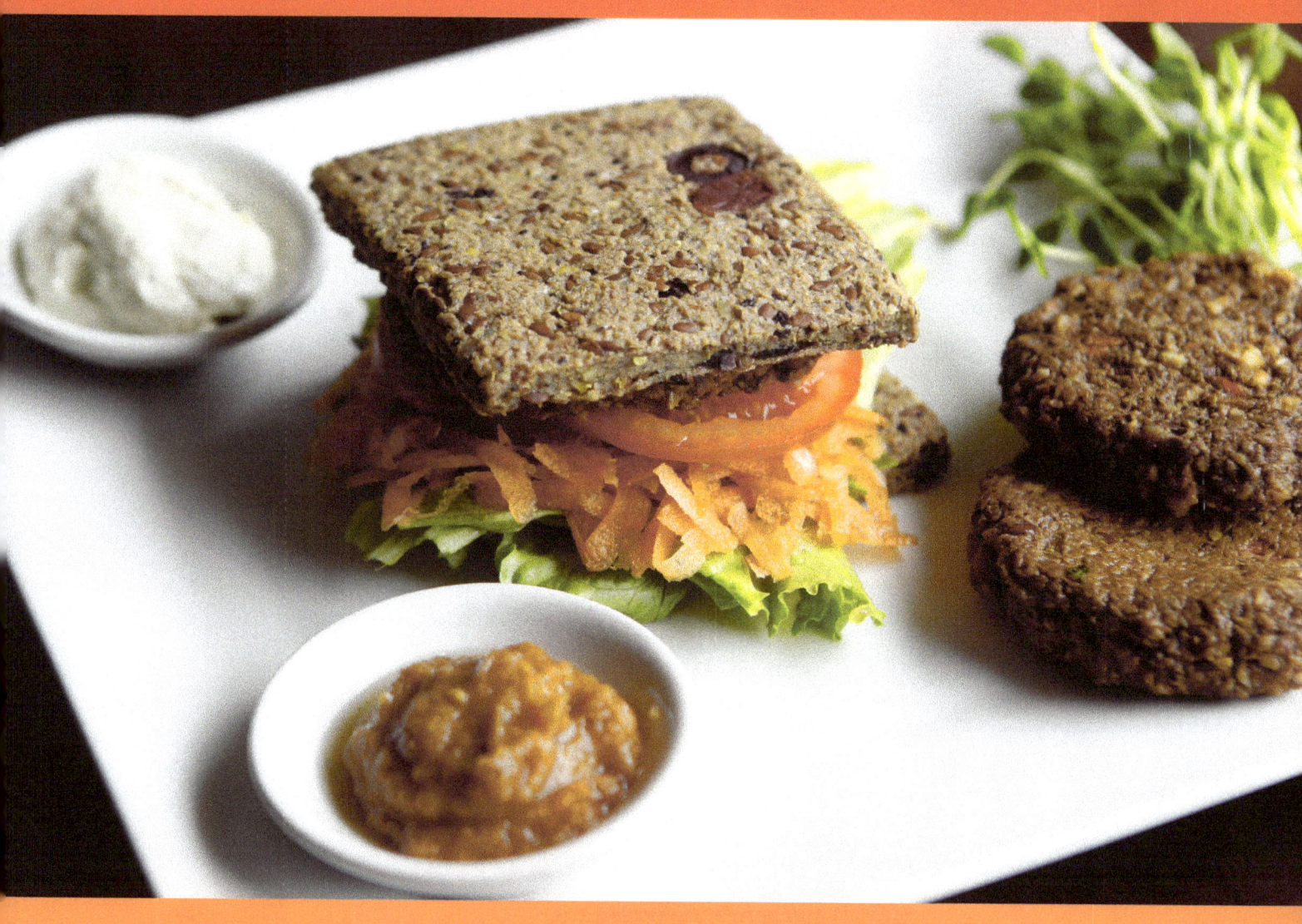

These burgers and patties are satisfying, healthy and easy to make. You can store most of these for at least a week in the fridge and use them as a quick, filling treat to satisfy a hungry tummy. If you are not following a completely raw diet, you can grill until golden in the oven on a low heat or bake quickly in a pan with a little raw coconut oil.

sun burgers ...
makes 6 to 8 patties

1 cup of walnuts
1 cup of almonds
1 cup of flaxseeds (soaked)
1 cup of portabella mushrooms, chopped
1 carrot, grated
½ red capsicum
2 garlic cloves
1 tablespoon of genmai miso
4 tablespoons of tamari
a handful of coriander
water to blend

Puree nuts, flaxseeds, mushrooms, carrots, garlic, capsicum and slowly add in miso, tamari, coriander and enough water to form a dough like texture. Form into little balls and squash into pattie shapes on a dehydrator tray. Dehydrate at 145 F or 62 C for one hour, then reduce to 115 F or 46 C, cooking until ready or golden on one side. Flip over, place back on mesh screens and dehydrate on the other side for 2 more hours or until ready.

quick tip ...

The burgers in this section are dehydrated to ensure that no enzymes or nutrients are destroyed with heat. If you do not have a dehydrator or you don't wish to go completely raw yet, try quickly pan frying burgers in a little coconut oil to cook or grill in the oven on a low temperature until ready. To power up your burgers with extra nutrition, replace any nuts or seeds for their sprouted versions.

curried nut burgers
makes 4 to 6 patties

1 cup of almonds
1 cup of sunflower seeds
1 cup of pre-soaked flaxseeds
1 cup of portabella mushrooms, chopped
1 small carrot, grated
1 small red capsicum
2 garlic cloves
4 tablespoons of tamari or Bragg's
1 teaspoon of Celtic salt
1 tablespoon of shiro miso paste
4 fresh curry leaves or 2 tablespoons of curry powder
2 to 4 tablespoons of sesame oil
2 pitted medjool dates
½ lemon, juiced

Soak nuts and seeds for 4 to 6 hours. Drain and puree with garlic, mushrooms, carrot, capsicum, miso, dates, tamari, curry powder, lemon juice and oil. Form into small patties and place on a dehydrator tray and cook at 145 F or 62 C for 1 hour, reduce temperature to 115 F or 46 C until golden brown. Flip over & dehydrate on the other side for another 2 hrs. If you are not following completely raw, put a little coconut oil in a pan and brown on both sides or heat under a grill

spicy turmeric tofu fillets

This is a wonderful flavoursome and spicy coating that can be used for tofu, tempeh, vegetables or any type of fish

4 to 6 slices of fresh tofu, tempeh or thinly sliced vegetables
¼ cup of organic, extra-virgin coconut oil
2 tablespoons of paprika
2 tablespoons of turmeric
2 teaspoons of onion powder
1 teaspoon of cayenne
1 teaspoon of dried coriander
½ teaspoon of ground cumin
1 teaspoon of Celtic salt
fresh lemon

Combine all dry seasonings in a shallow bowl and mix well. Place coconut oil in a shallow bowl. Dip tofu slices in coconut oil and then coat with dry seasoning mix. Place on a dehydrator tray and cook until golden brown on both sides. Sprinkle a little chopped mint, rosemary or coriander on the top when finished and squeeze with fresh lemon juice. Spicy tofu fillets can also be blended and used in lettuce wraps, rice paper rolls and tomato cups.

raw thai fish cakes ...
makes 8 to 10 fish cakes

Soak nuts and seeds for a few hours or overnight. Rinse and drain well. Blend 1 cup of soaked flaxseeds with the rest of the ingredients until you get a nice dough texture. Shape into little patties and dehydrate at a slightly higher temperature for one hour, then reduce to 115 F or 46 C until dry on one side. Remove and flip over and place on a mesh screen to dehydrate on the other side. These are so delicious – they taste exactly like thai fish cakes, minus the fish.

1 cup of portabello mushrooms, chopped
1 cup of almonds (soaked for a few hours)
1 cup of pre-soaked flaxseeds
⅛ cup of black sesame seeds
2 red chillies, diced
1 small carrot, chopped in chunks or grated
3 to 4 sun-dried tomatoes
2 kaffir lime leaves, finely chopped
a handful of scallions, spring onions or chives
1 inch chunk of ginger, chopped
1 inch chunk of galangal, chopped
2 to 3 garlic cloves, chopped
a handful of coriander, chopped
1 teaspoon of Celtic salt or 2 tablespoons of Bragg's

burrito cups ...

oriental burrito ...

burritos
4 cabbage or lettuce leaves, green or purple

filling
2 cups of bok choy, tat soi or rocket
1 cup of bean sprouts
2 tablespoons of extra virgin sesame oil
a little tamari
2 limes, squeezed
1 cup of nut meat (recipe in 'Condiments, Spreads and Dips')
1 serve of Asian guacamole (recipe in 'Condiments, Spreads and Dips')

Toss chopped tat soi, bok choy or rocket with bean sprouts in sesame oil, tamari and lime juice. Put aside for ten minutes. When ready, place in the bottom of each burrito cup. Top with nutty meat, Asian guacamole and fresh lime juice. A yummy Asian burrito with a twist.

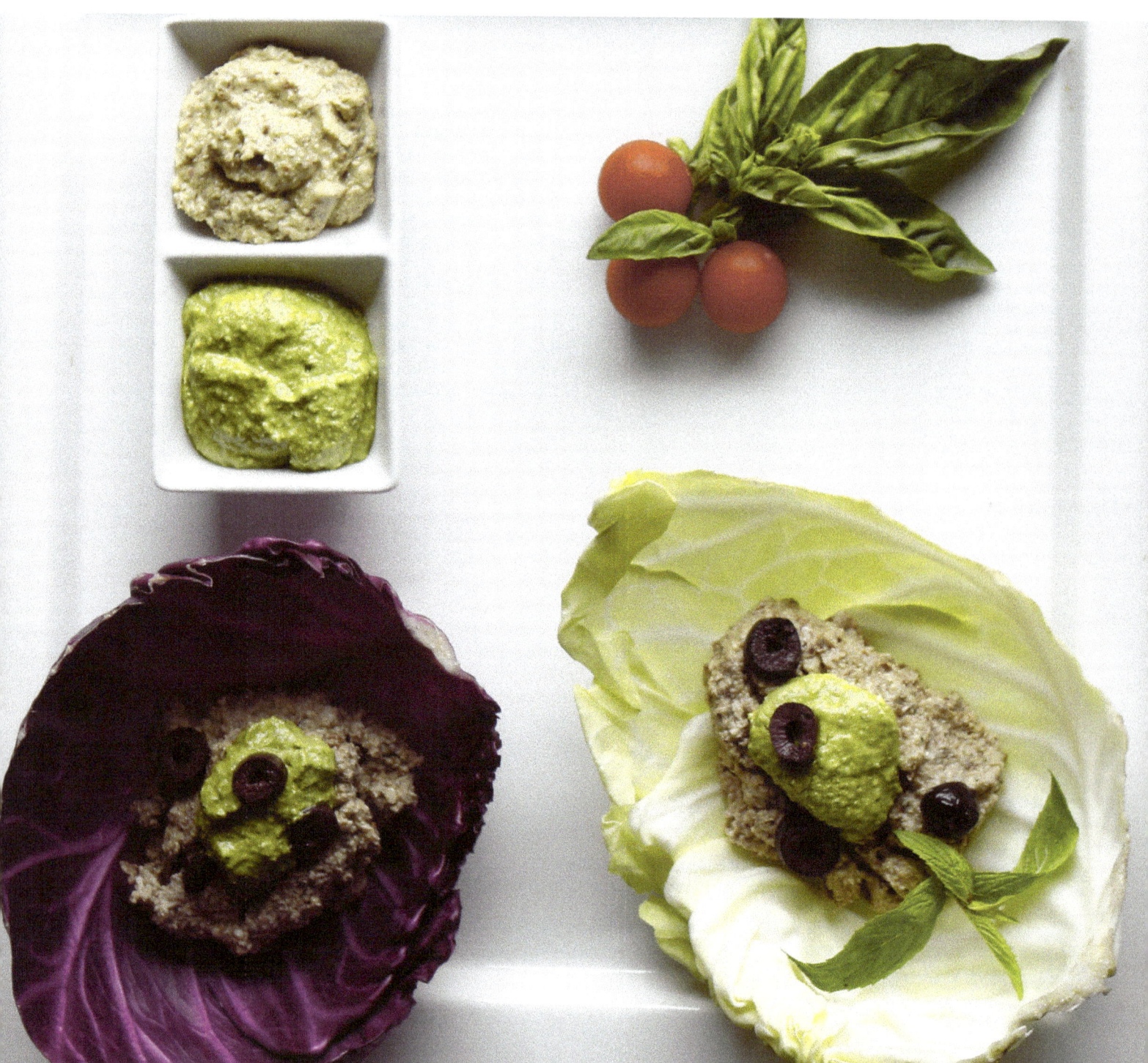

southern burrito ...

I love to use lettuce or cabbage leaves instead of corn burritos to make yummy, but healthy wraps. Green or purple cabbage leaves peel off easily to make fantastic vegetable cups that you can fill with mock cheese, salsa, guacamole and other delicious ingredients. You can leave the leaves open or roll up and put a toothpick through to make a burrito type creation. These are amazing for dinner parties - they look spectacular and your friends will be surprised at just how yummy these taste.

burritos
4 cabbage leaves, purple or green or both

filling
2 cups of baby spinach
1 corn cob, shredded
2 tablespoons of extra virgin olive oil
a pinch of Celtic salt
1 cup of nutty meat (recipe in 'Condiments, spreads and dips')
1 serve of spicy raw tomato salsa (recipe in 'Condiments, Spreads and Dips')

Toss spinach leaves and corn with olive oil and Celtic salt and put aside. Place into the bottom of each leaf cup. Spread with nutty meat and spicy tomato salsa. This is a delicious burrito with a healthy twist. You can even put some yummy guacamole on top with a squeeze of lemon juice and fresh paprika.

mediterranean burrito ...

burritos
4 cabbage or lettuce leaves, green or purple

filling
1 cup of rocket leaves
1 cup of baby spinach
1 red capsicum
2 tablespoons of extra virgin olive oil
a pinch of Celtic salt
1 cup of nutty meat (recipe in 'Condiments, Spreads and Dips')
1 serve of basic pesto (recipe in 'Condiments, Spreads and Dips')
1 lemon, juiced
a little pure balsamic vinegar

Toss rocket and baby spinach with olive oil and Celtic salt and put aside for five minutes. Place into the bottom of each cabbage or lettuce cup. Top with nutty meat and basic pesto. If you have made a delicious mock cheese, put this on top also. Squeeze lemon juice on top. This is a yummy Mediterranean burrito with a healthy twist.

sushi rolls (rice free) ...
makes around 12 pieces

mock rice
2 cups of macadamia or cashews
(pre-soaked for a few hours to soften)
a little lemon juice
1 clove of garlic
1 teaspoon of minced or grated ginger
a few mint leaves
¼ yellow onion
2 teaspoons of brown rice vinegar
a little raw honey or
yacon or agave

insides
cucumber sticks
avocado
carrot slices

Put nuts into a blender with lemon juice, garlic, ginger, mint, onion, rice vinegar and natural sweetener – pulse the mix to keep grainy and not too watery. Spread a thin layer across a nori sheet leaving one inch free from your far end. Place vegetable sticks, avocado, pickled ginger and any other ingredient lengthwise in the middle. Use the bamboo mat to roll up the nori sheets. Slice into sushi pieces and serve with tamari and wasabi. A great snack for parties!

cauliflower sushi ...
makes around 12 pieces

1 large cauliflower floret
2 teaspoons of brown rice vinegar
2 teaspoons of raw honey or agave

insides
cucumber sticks
avocado
carrot slices etc

Put cauliflower into a blender and blend until it looks like rice – keep grainy. Then mix with rice vinegar, raw honey or agave until you get a sweet rice taste. Spread a layer of the mix over your nori sheet leaving one inch from the end to roll properly. Put your fillings inside – carrot sticks, cucumber sticks, snow pea sprouts, avocado etc and do a thin layer of wasabi mayonnaise. Roll up with a bamboo mat and slice the sushi into pieces. Serve with tamari and wasabi

pickled ginger ...
makes 1 jar

1 large chunk of ginger, sliced thinly
4 tablespoons of brown rice vinegar
2 lemons, juiced
1 to 2 tablespoons of pure cane
or palm sugar
⅛ teaspoon of natural citric acid
a little purified water

Cut ginger into very thin slices. Mix together brown rice vinegar, sugar, lemon juice and water. Put this liquid into a glass jar and add ginger to the mix. Add the citric acid at the end to preserve the ginger for longer. This is ready to eat in two days and will keep in the fridge for weeks

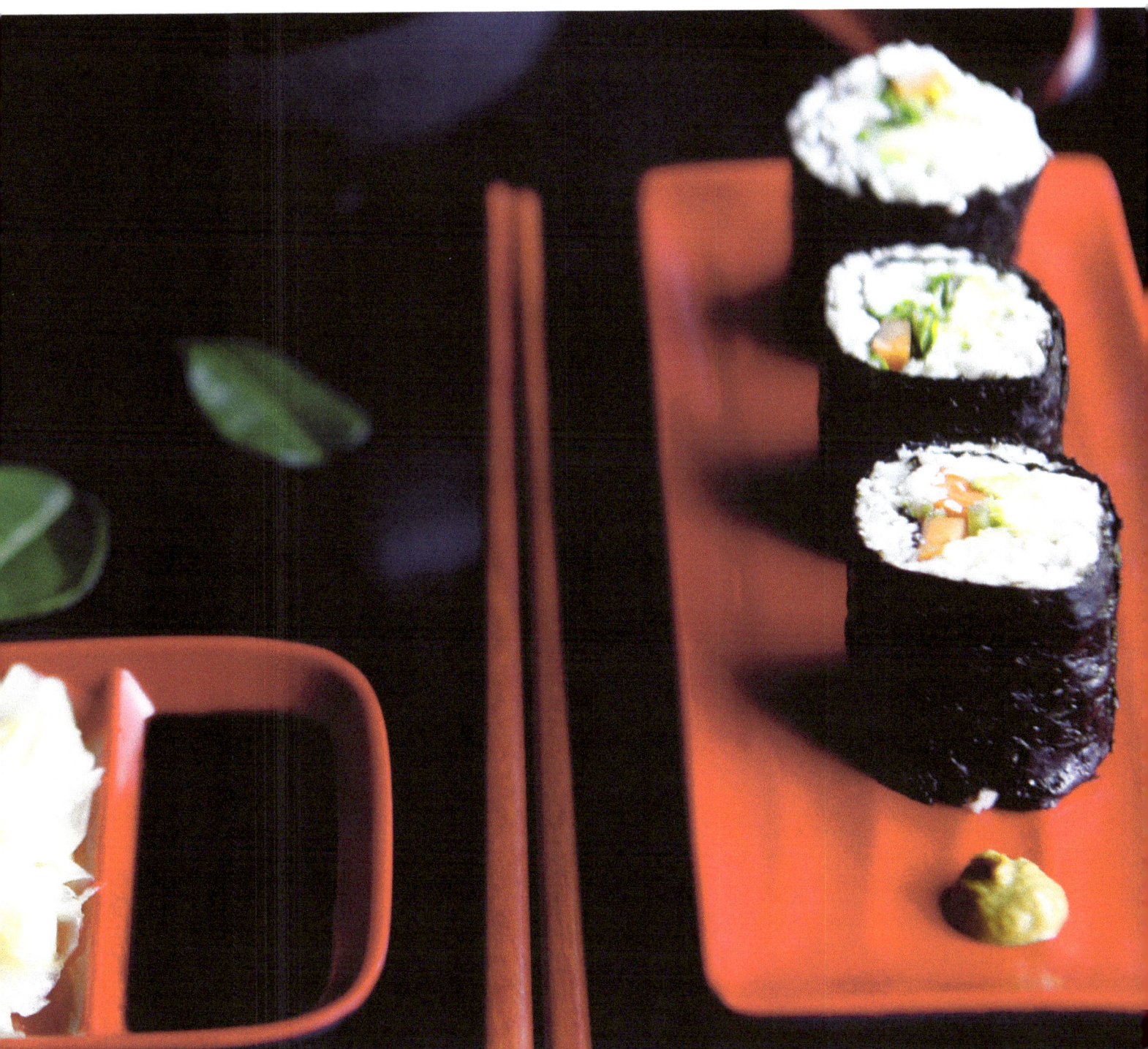

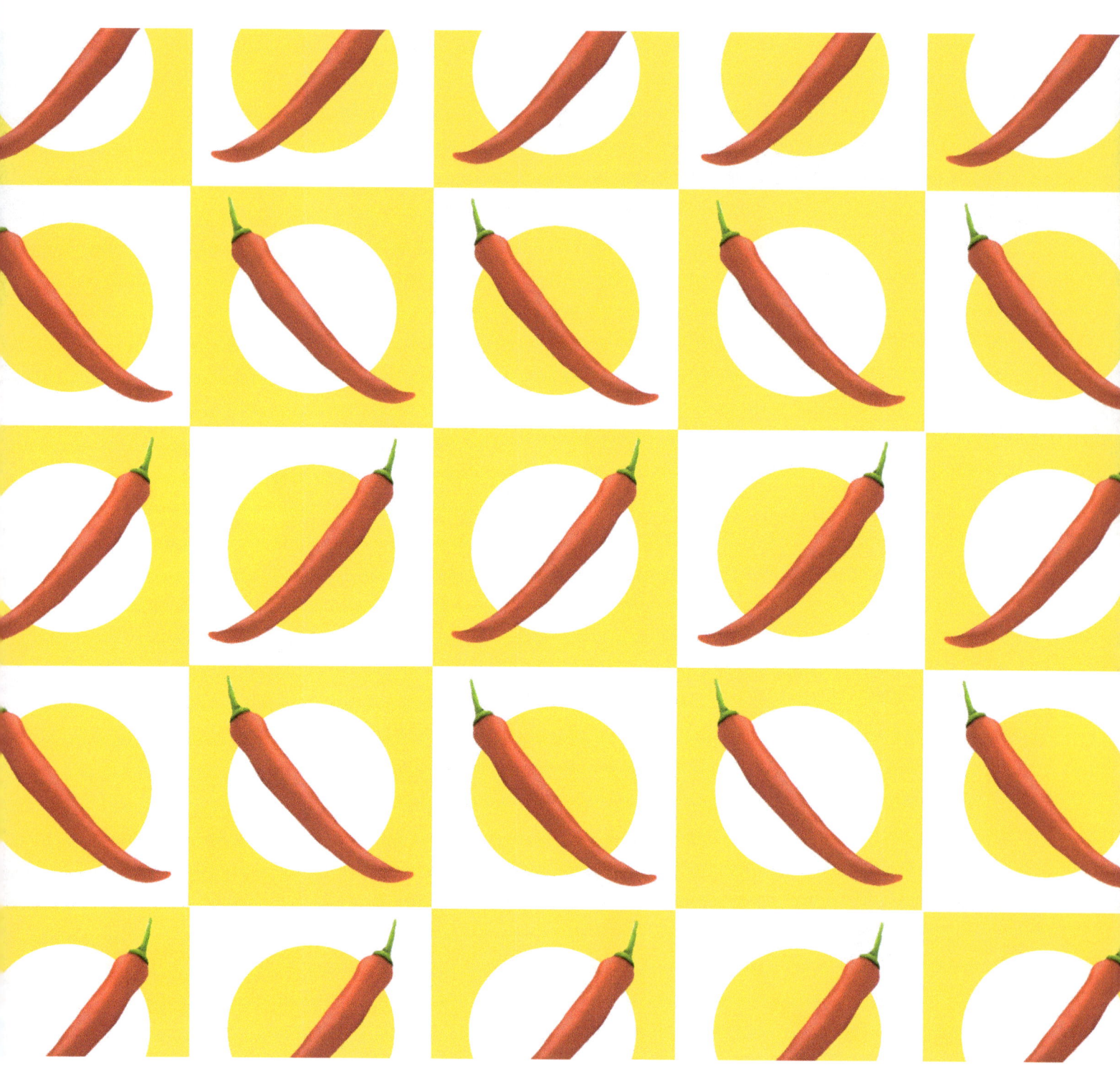

curry in a hurry ...

thai red curry with noodles ...
serves 3

noodles
4 zucchini or squash
2 carrots
2 cups of bean sprouts
1 coconut, shred the meat
3 tablespoons of tamari or Bragg's
3 tablespoons of sesame oil

curry sauce
1 block of firm, organic tofu (optional)
½ small onion, chopped
2 garlic cloves
2 tablespoons of olive oil
3 tablespoons of pitted dates or 2 pitted medjool dates
3 teaspoons of red curry paste or leaves
2 kaffir lime leaves
2 limes, juiced
4 tablespoons of tamari or Bragg's
½ cup of coriander
1 cup of purified water or almond milk

To make the noodles, turn zucchini and carrots into noodle shapes with a spiralizer or spirooli. Place in a bowl with bean sprouts, shredded coconut, tamari or Bragg's and sesame oil. Set aside.

To make the sauce, process onion, dates, garlic, red curry paste or leaves, lime leaves, olive oil, coriander, tamari and lime juice. Add a little water and tofu – pulse keeping the tofu grainy. Place noodles in three bowls and top with the curry sauce. If you want your curry hot, heat up slightly on a stove keeping below 115 F or 46 C. When ready, sprinkle with chopped chilli and fresh lime juice. If you don't eat tofu, replace with cauliflower.

tibetan antioxidant curry
serves 3

½ onion, chopped
2 cups of cauliflower or broccoli florets
1 cup of fresh green peas
2 carrots, chopped
½ cup of goji berries
1 green chilli or (1 tsp or minced chilli paste)
2 teaspoons of mild curry powder
1 teaspoon of turmeric (fresh or powdered)
1 tablespoon of grated ginger
1 teaspoon of Celtic salt
1 teaspoon of cumin
2 tablespoons of fresh coriander
1 lime, juiced
1 cup of hot water
a few cardamom seeds or pods (optional)

In a food processor mix together onion, goji berries, green chilli, lime juice, ginger, turmeric, cumin, cauliflower, carrots and coriander with a little warm water. When you have a nice texture, stir in green peas and broccoli. Serve alone or with dehydrated quinoa or sprouted rice. If you are not following completely raw, serve with red quinoa or brown rice.

sprouted dhal
serves 2 to 3

1 cup of sprouted lentils
1 tablespoon of curry powder
½ teaspoon of ginger
1 to 2 cloves of garlic
½ teaspoon of cinnamon
½ teaspoon of turmeric
¼ teaspoon of Celtic salt
3 tablespoons of pure coconut meat or milk
½ red capsicum
water

Blend sprouted lentils in a blender until just coarse. Add curry powder, ginger, cinnamon, turmeric, red capsicum, garlic and Celtic salt with a little water and coconut milk. Warm slightly or eat cool. A spicy taste sensation.

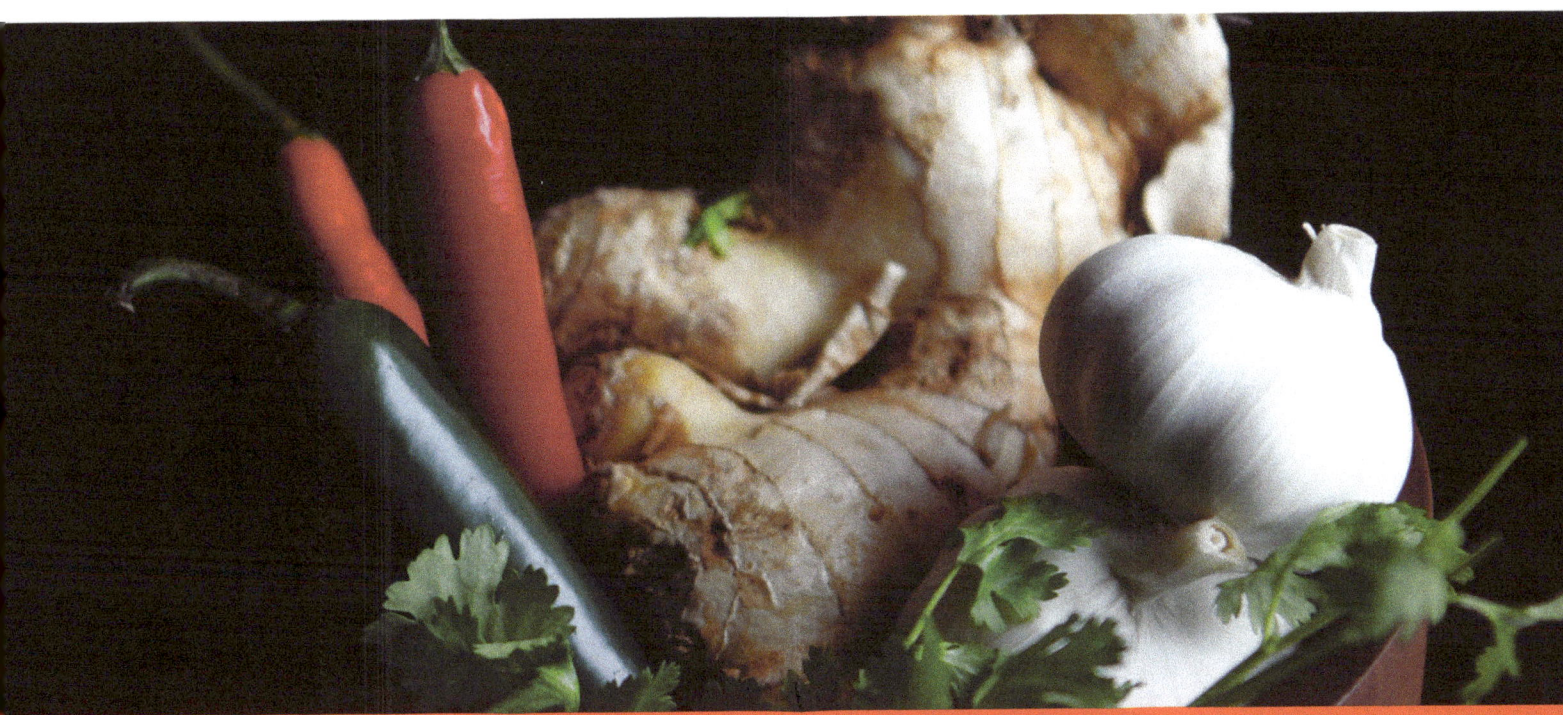

more mains to die for ...

peppered garlic tofu ...
makes 10 to 12 slices

Cut tofu into thin slices. In a blender mix grated carrot, lime juice, oil, almonds or pistachio, coriander, black peppercorns, natural sweetener and tamari until you get a slightly chunky mix. Put this mix into a bowl and place tofu fillets in the bowl to marinate for around twenty minutes. Place marinated tofu fillets onto teflex sheets in the dehydrator. Cook at 145 F or 62 C for one hour, then reduce to 105 F or 46 C and heat until golden brown. Squeeze lemon juice and a little tamari on each steak before eating. These are also yummy in sunflower bread or lettuce cups.

1 small block of organic, GMO free tofu
1 carrot, grated
1 lime, squeezed
1 garlic clove
¼ cup of organic sesame oil or coconut oil
2 tablespoons of almonds or pistachio's (pre-soaked)
¼ cup of coriander
4 tablespoons of black peppercorns
1 teaspoon of agave or yacon
4 tablespoons of tamari

mediterranean tomato cups ...

makes 6 tomato cups

filling
- a small handful of black olives, pitted
- ½ cucumber, finely chopped
- 2 celery sticks, finely chopped
- 2 spring onions, finely chopped
- ¼ cup of fresh parsley, finely chopped
- ¼ cup of fresh basil, finely chopped
- 2 garlic cloves, minced
- ¼ cup of pine nuts
- 1 lemon, juiced
- 2 tablespoons of olive oil
- ½ teaspoon of Celtic salt

tomato cups
6 medium tomatoes

Cut tomatoes in half and scoop out the pulp. Add the pulp to the rest of the finely diced ingredients. Mix well in a bowl and fill the tomato halves with the mixture. Eat the tomato cups raw or dehydrate at 115 F or 46 C until golden brown.

---

stuffed bell pepper mushrooms ...

makes 15 to 20 mushrooms

red capsicum mix
- ½ red capsicum, chopped
- ½ cup of sunflower seeds (pre-soaked)
- ¼ cup of raw almonds (pre-soaked)
- 1 celery, chopped
- 2 garlic cloves
- 1 teaspoon of Celtic salt
- 1 teaspoon of turmeric or onion powder
- ½ teaspoon of cayenne pepper
- ½ teaspoon of cumin
- 4 tablespoons of fresh parsley or mint, chopped
- 1 lemon, juiced
- 2 teaspoons of agave nectar or 5 dates (pitted)
- 1/3 cup of organic macadamia or olive oil

mushroom cups
15 to 20 large button or baby bella mushrooms

Process all of the ingredients, except mushrooms in a food processor and slowly add oil until creamy. Remove stems from the mushrooms and fill with red capsicum mix. Put sliced olives on top of mix. Put into the dehydrator and set temperature at 115 F or 46C. Heat until they are golden brown. Squeeze lemon juice on top before serving.

creamy olive dip in vegetable cups

makes 4 to 8 vegetable cups

Process avocado, olives, salt, cumin, onion, garlic, ginger, lemon juice and dates with oil. Either leave chunky by pulsing the mix or make creamy, depending on which texture you like.

To make the vege cups, slice the top off capsicum or tomatoes, scoop the insides out and place the olive dip inside. Sprinkle with cayenne or paprika and dehydrate for a hot treat in winter. If you do not have a dehydrator, heat up under a grill keeping below 115F or 46C.

vegetable cups

4 tomatoes or
8 large lettuce leaves or
4 small red capsicum

olive dip

½ cup of pitted black olives
1 ½ avocadoes
¼ cup of olive oil or flaxseed oil
1 purple onion
2 garlic cloves
2 teaspoons of cumin
2 teaspoons of grated or minced ginger
1 to 2 fresh lemons, juiced
1 teaspoon of Celtic salt
3 to 5 pitted medjool dates
1 teaspoon of jalapeno
(optional – if you want a little extra spice)

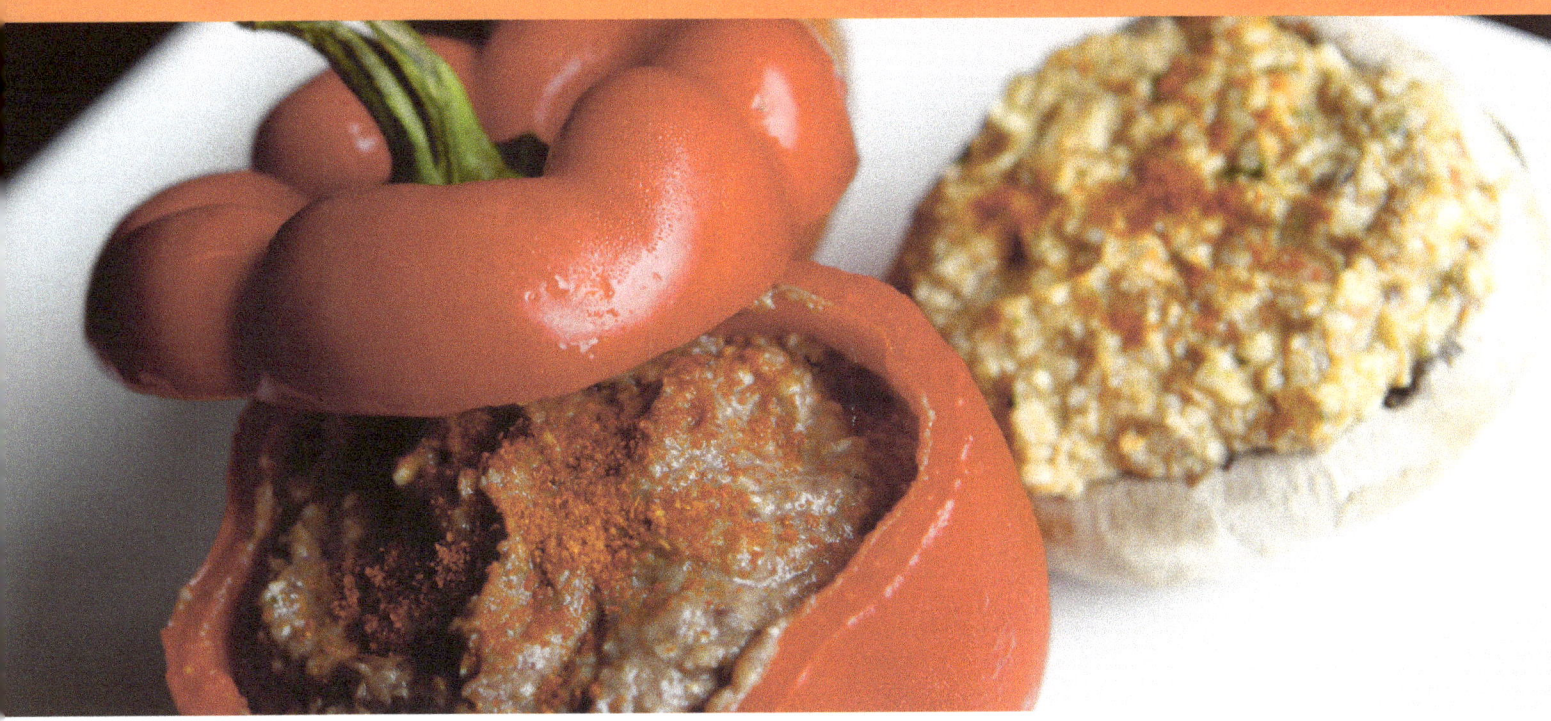

eggplant pizzas ...
makes around 20 small pizza's

base
2 large eggplants

topping
**1 cup of sesame seeds (pre-soaked for 3 hours)
⅛ cup of walnuts (pre-soaked for 3 hours)
2 garlic cloves
2 tomatoes
a handful of fresh mint
a handful of fresh basil
1 lemon
2 tablespoons of tamari
4 tablespoons of olive oil
2 teaspoons of agave or 3 pitted dates
tomato salsa
(refer to recipe in 'condiments, spreads and dips')**

De-skin eggplant, then cut into thin circles. Process garlic, tomato, nuts and seeds, mint, basil, lime juice, dates, tamari and olive oil. Spread the filling ingredients onto the eggplant circles and add a layer of salsa. You can also add a little 'pizza pete' cheese if you have made this up. Either lay flat in the shape of a pizza or fold in half and hold using a toothpick, just like a burrito.

Dehydrate at 145 F or 62 C for 1 hour, then reduce to 115 F or 46 C until golden brown. If you don't have a dehydrator, you can warm in the oven or under a grill until ready.

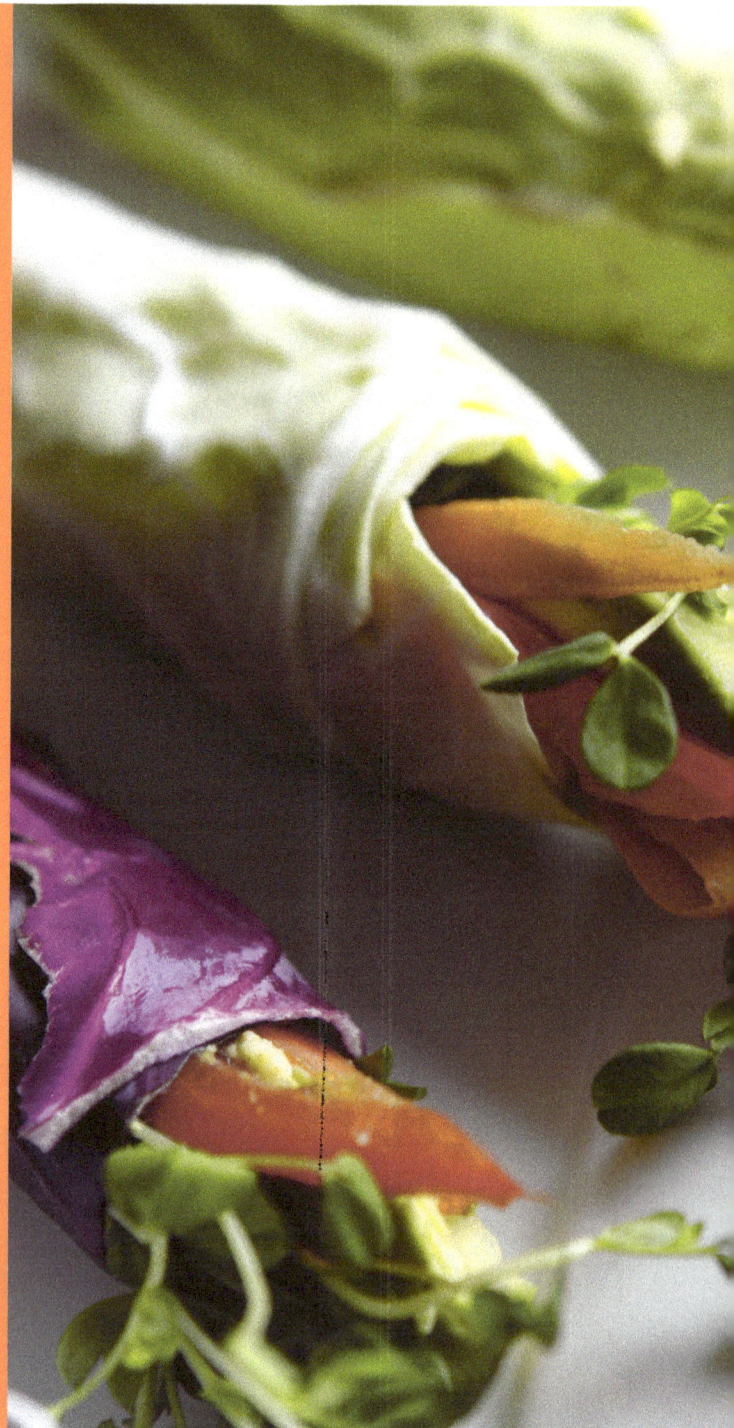

vietnamese lettuce or cabbage rolls ...
makes 4 to 6 lettuce rolls

cabbage rolls
4 to 8 large cabbage or lettuce leaves

filling
1 cucumber, remove skin and cut into thin strips
1 carrot, cut into thin strips
1 avocado, cut into thin strips
1 bunch of snow pea sprouts
1 bunch of bean sprouts

dipping sauce
¼ cup of chopped almonds
3 tablespoons of natural fish sauce
(made from anchovies – use Bragg's
or Tamari if you are a vegetarian)
2 limes, juiced
1 red chilli, finely chopped
3 tablespoons of rice vinegar
1 teaspoon of agave
¼ cup of mint
¼ cup of coriander

Get a large lettuce and remove the leaves, cut into square shapes or leave natural. Fill with strips of cucumber, carrot, avocado, snow pea sprouts and bean sprouts. To make the dipping sauce, blend lime juice, fish sauce or tamari, rice vinegar, agave, chilli, chopped almonds, mint and coriander. Leave slightly chunky and pour a little over the filling. Then roll up lettuce or cabbage leaves and use a toothpick or carrot stick to hold. Simply delicious!

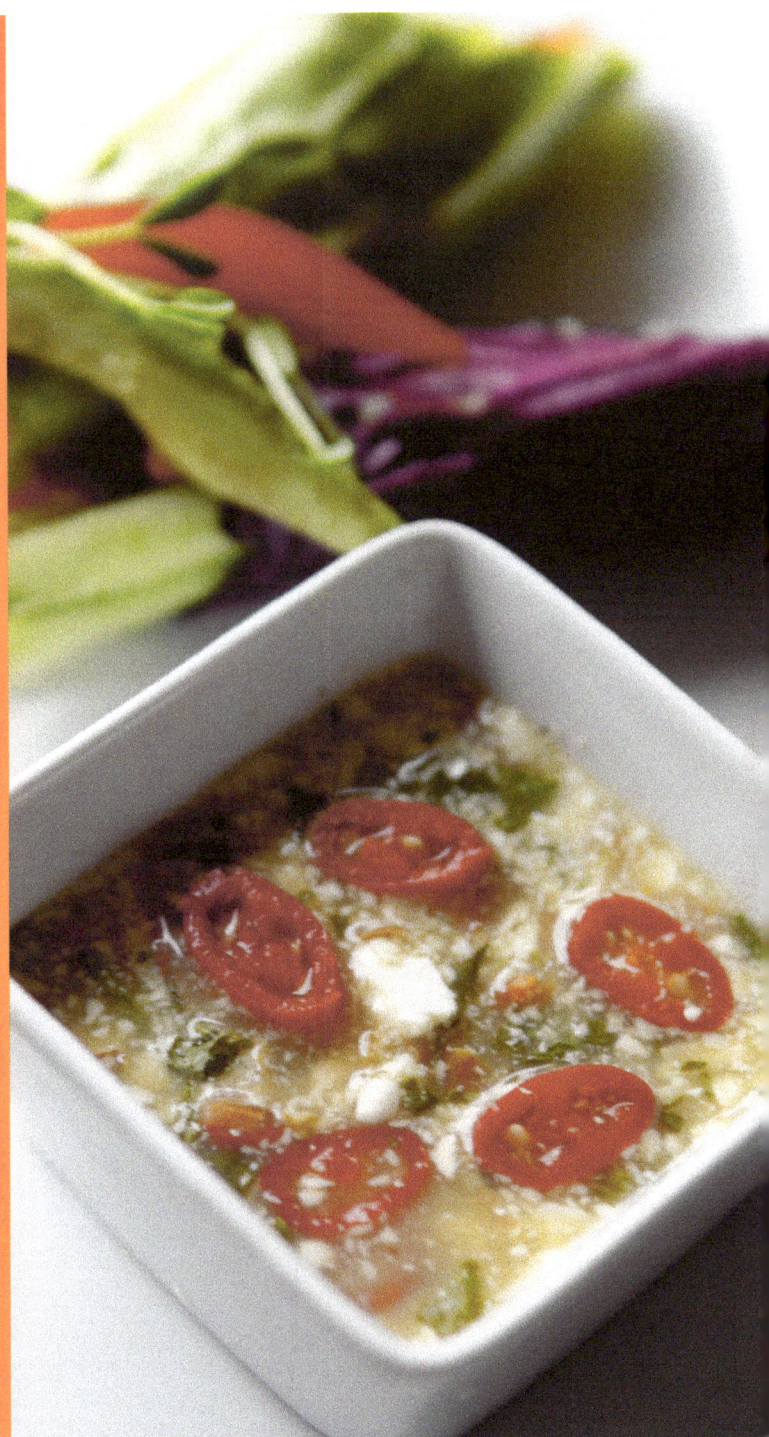

Creamy Treats and Ice-Dreams
Raspberry Cinnamon Cream
Hazelnut Vanilla Ice Dream
Strawberry Chocolate Mousse

Cakes and Pies
Passionfruit Cheesecake
Double Choc Beet Cake
Blueberry Cheesecake
Raw Chocolate Pecan Pie

Not so Naughty Treats ...

Super Slices and Chocolate Indulgence
Decadent Chocolate Slice
Superfood Chocolate Truffles
Chocolate to Die For
Nutty Choc Balls
Fig Fudge
Vanilla Goji Balls

When I make 'sweet treats' I always opt for natural fruits or plant sources as a natural sweetener. A huge intake of sugar does more harm to the human body than nearly any substance. One teaspoon of refined sugar per day can suppress immunity for two to three hours and more than three teaspoons per day can suppress immunity for at least half a day. Excess intake of sugar not only causes severe swings in blood glucose levels that can lead to mood swings, diabetes, weight gain and hypoglycaemia, it is also responsible for countless other health ailments. Below are some of the reasons why it is better to eat natural, sugar-free sweets over high sugared desserts.

the danger of WHITE POISON ...
A high sugar intake causes ...

Headaches and migraines
Poor vision and eye problems
Suppressed immunity
Hyperactivity, behavioural problems, poor learning and decreased attention span
High cholesterol and triglycerides that can clog up arteries
Depression, irritability, anxiety and mood swings
Reduced sensitivity to insulin causing metabolic syndrome, weight gain and diabetes
Damage to DNA
Mineral excretion leading to osteoporosis and acidity problems
Haemorrhoids and constipation
PMS symptoms
Poor release of growth hormone, stunting growth in children
Kidney stones and high uric acid levels
Increased risk of strokes and heart attacks
Low energy and poor stress resistance
High fat content within the liver causing fatty liver
And many more.....

It is important to read labels very carefully, as sugar is cleverly disguised under names like beet, grape or date sugar, corn syrup, corn syrup solids, high-fructose corn syrup, dextrose, dehydrated cane juice or cane juice crystals, ethyl maltol, fructose, glucose, glucose solids, golden syrup, processed honey, invert sugar, lactose, malt syrup, maltodextrin, maltose, mannitol, sorbitol, processed maple syrup, raw sugar, rice syrup and sucrose.

The more we understand about the danger of 'refined and fake sugar substances', the more it makes sense to switch to natural, antioxidant rich sugar alternatives found in nature. Not only do they contain natural sugars which are healthier for your pancreas, most of these also contain healing phytonutrients to improve health and immune defences. By choosing 'natural sweeteners' you are not only satisfying your sweet needs, but also increasing the healing potential of the foods that you eat. For anyone on a strictly 'SUGAR-FREE' diet, replace any of the natural sweeteners given in the recipes below with raw and unrefined sources of stevia, unprocessed xylitol, erythritol, yacon syrup and a small amount of medjool dates.

which natural sweetener do i choose?

There are hundreds of so called 'natural sweetener's' on the market, all claiming to have the lowest glycemic index and sugar content with the highest nutrition. While all of these claims seem incredible, are they actually true? Below are some of my favourite natural sweeteners and their positive and negative attributes in sweetening dishes.

Stevia is one of my favourite natural sweeteners and in fact one of the healthiest. It has no calories, no sugar content and does not cause any spikes in glucose, making it great for diabetics or anyone on a cancer fighting program. Stevia is up to 300 times sweeter than sugar and its only disadvantage is its slightly bitter taste and in some people it can cause diarrhea or stomach cramps, when used in excess. Only two to four drops of stevia will equate to one teaspoon of normal sugar in taste. Always look for an unprocessed form of stevia.

Erythritol is another good option. This is a 'natural sugar alcohol' taken from certain fruits and vegetables. It is 60% as sweet as sugar and contains only 4 grams of carbohydrates and 4 grams of sugar per one teaspoon. This makes it a very healthy alternative for sweetening dishes and it creates no gastrointestinal upsets.

Xylitol is a natural sugar alcohol that was originally derived from the Scandinavian birch tree. It is as sweet as sugar, yet it does not cause any spiking in glucose like sugar. It also has healing properties, working to strengthen mucous membrane linings helping with sinusitis, rhinitis and ear, nose and throat problems. However, it is important to beware when buying xylitol as most of this is now made from modified corn starch. Look for a pure xylitol made from birch trees or organic corn.

Medjool dates are a natural fruit that is rich in fibre, B vitamins, minerals and antioxidants. One date supplies 16 grams of sugar and 18 grams of carbohydrates. Even though its fructose content is quite high, the other nutrients found within this healthy fruit help to digest the fructose without causing any spikes in blood sugar. With medjool dates, you only need to use a small amount to sweeten dishes.

Lucuma powder is found in lots of my vanilla and chocolate recipes. It is a native Peruvian fruit that is a wonderful source of carbohydrates, minerals, antioxidants, beta-carotene and B vitamins. It does not cause any spikes in blood sugar, making it a perfect addition for anyone who wants a healthy sweetener.

Yacon syrup is extracted from the native South American yacon plant. It is a brilliant source of iron and a natural prebiotic that can improve digestive function. It contains half the calories of honey and is much lower in glycemic index than most natural sweeteners, running at only one. It causes no spikes in blood sugar and is a good choice to sweeten raw food desserts and smoothies. To ensure it stays raw, it must be produced at temperatures below 40 degrees C. It has a caramel-like molasses flavour and is as sweet as sugar, so use in the same proportion as you would agave or honey. It is thick, sticky and can add moisture to dishes.

cont over page ...

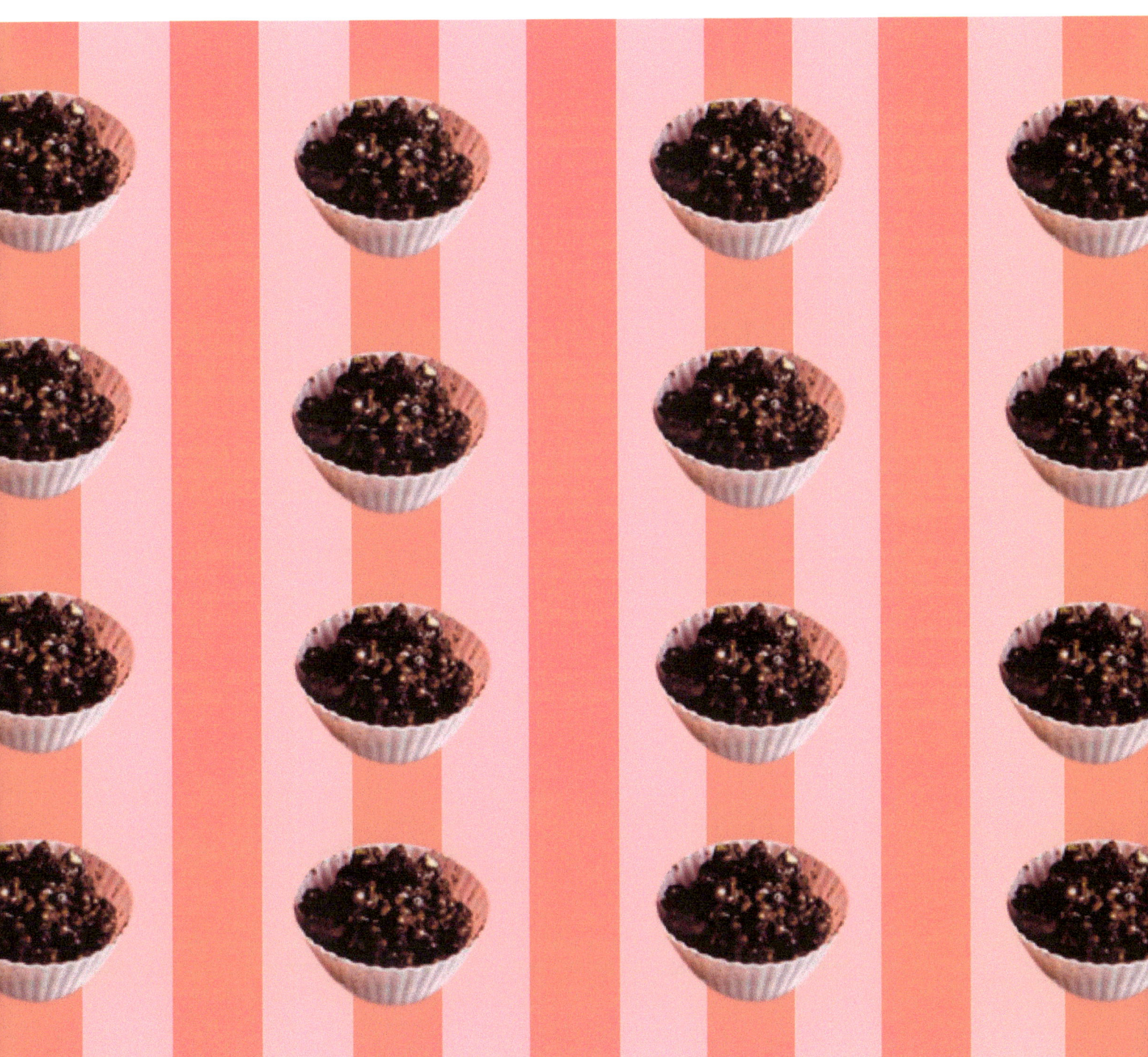

Rapadura sugar is evaporated sugar cane juice. It normally takes very little heat to process this sugar, which allows most of the vitamins and minerals to be preserved. Rapadura contains fructose, glucose and sucrose making it much easier to digest than normal sugar. One teaspoon converts to 4 grams of sugar. It should still be used extremely moderately, as a high intake can affect your insulin balance.

Coconut palm sugar is taken from the nectar of the coconut palm. It is then boiled lowering the moisture content, allowing it to become solid. Once cool it is then granulated. Its glycemic index is 35, making it lower than cane sugar, honey or agave. It contains 12 amino acids and fair amounts of potassium, magnesium and phosphorous. It is a healthier alternative to rapadura, but should still be used moderately.

Agave syrup is a healthier alternative to sugar, that is, if you can find a raw, natural agave that isn't exposed to high heats during processing. Agave syrup is derived from the Mexican agave plant. It is primarily 90% fructose with glucose. Most of the agave products found in the stores are highly processed and contain hydrolyzed high fructose inulin syrup. If you can find an unprocessed, organic and reliable source of natural agave, then it can definitely be used moderately without causing weight gain, diabetes and heart problems.

Honey, when found in a raw and unprocessed form, contains 17 grams of carbohydrates, with 16 grams of this being pure fructose and glucose. Honey is much sweeter than normal sugar, so you can use less when making sweets. It is also a great source of B vitamins, minerals and antioxidants. Because of its high calorie and sugar intake, it should still be used very moderately. When buying honey, only purchase raw honey.

Maple syrup is a moderate source of manganese, potassium, calcium, magnesium and zinc, B vitamins and amino acids. Most of the maple syrup found in the supermarkets is 20% maple syrup, combined with corn syrup, preservatives and colourings. Processed maple syrup also contains formaldehyde (an embalming agent) and lead. Maple syrup is almost 60% natural sugars, so like agave and raw honey it should still be used in moderation, otherwise it will contribute to weight gain, diabetes and other problems.

Even though I use raw honey, agave or other natural sweeteners in some of the recipes in this book, please feel free to replace these with healthier sweeteners like stevia, medjool dates, yacon or erythritol if you are on a low sugar or completely sugar free diet.

creamy treats and ice-dreams ...

To make any of the delicious mousses or creams below into ice-dreams, simply put the mixture through a slow extraction juicer or an ice-cream maker to get the perfect texture. Place in the freezer and enjoy when ready!

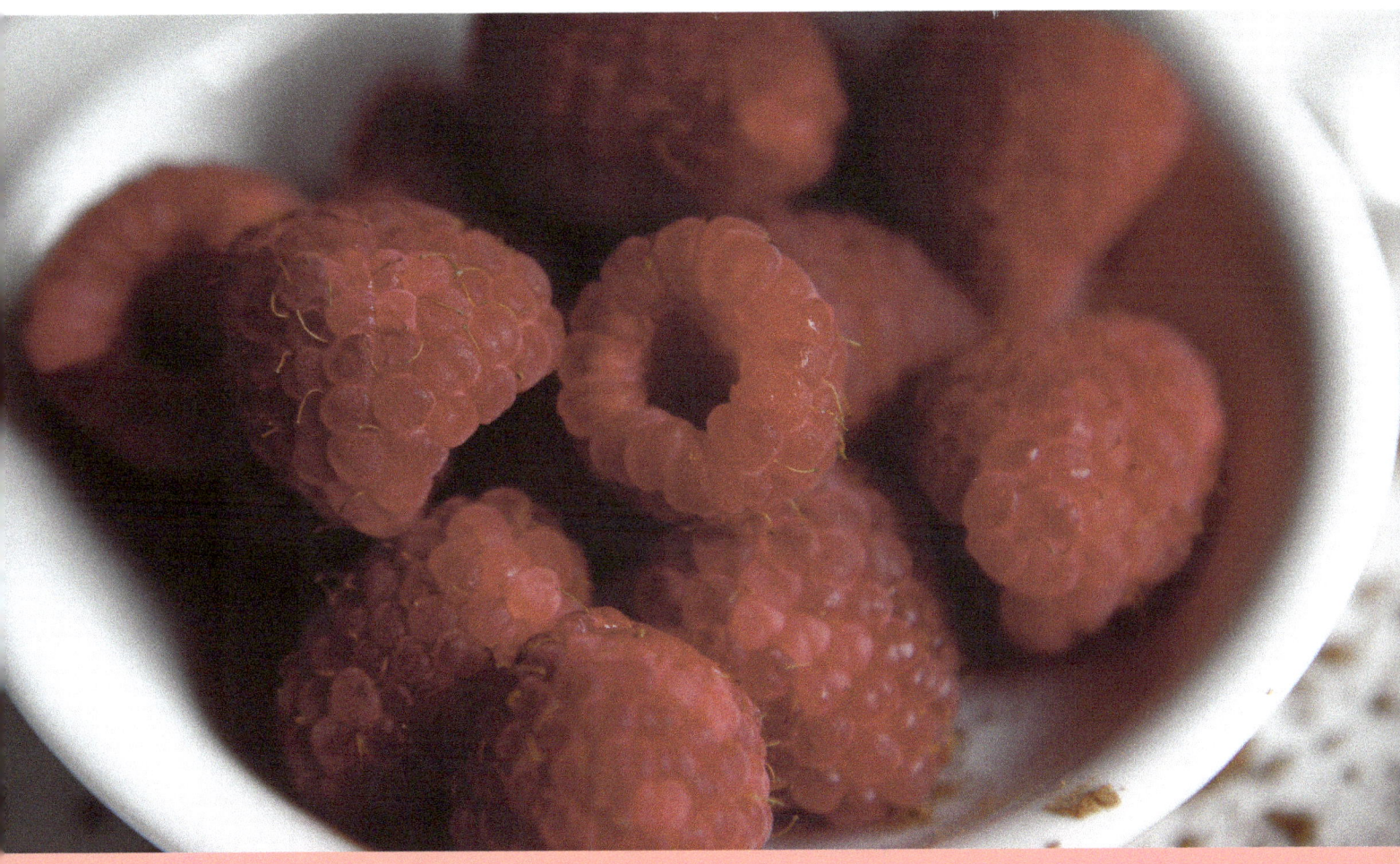

raspberry cinnamon cream ...
makes 2 to 3 glasses

Process the almonds and avocado with water until smooth. Add the natural sweetener, vanilla, cinnamon and raspberries. Blend until creamy and pour into glasses. Place in the fridge to set. This is a simple, delicious treat full of cancer fighting and heart-protective polyphenols.

2 cups of almonds (soaked or sprouted)
2 to 3 avocadoes
1 cup of raspberries or cherries (in season)
3 to 4 pitted medjool dates or 2 tbsp's of yacon syrup or 1 tsp or stevia or other
1 vanilla bean or 1 tablespoon of pure vanilla extract
1 teaspoon of cinnamon or a few cinnamon twigs
purified water

hazelnut vanilla ice dream
makes ¼ ice-cream tub

1 cup of cashews or macadamias
¼ cup of hazelnuts
½ cup of fresh coconut meat or coconut flakes
1 cup of nut milk
¼ cup of organic coconut oil
3 to 4 pitted medjool dates or 2 tablespoons of yacon syrup or other
2 teaspoons of pure vanilla extract
1 tablespoon of lucuma powder

Blend all of the ingredients in a food processor except hazelnuts, until creamy. Put the mix through an ice-cream maker or juicer to get the perfect texture. Crush your hazelnuts and mix through the ice-dream and then place in the freezer. To change the flavour of this ice dream, simply mix in strawberries, blueberries, peppermint oil, lemon rind or cacao pieces. Absolutely yummy! This will keep for weeks in the fridge. If you have time, pre-soak nuts

strawberry chocolate mousse
makes 3 to 4 sundae glasses

3 avocadoes
½ cup of raw cocoa powder
¼ cup of cacao powder
½ cup of extra virgin coconut oil
¼ cup of pitted dates (or ¼ cup of agave or yacon syrup)
¼ cup of fresh strawberries
1 teaspoon of lucuma powder (optional)
1 teaspoon of mesquite powder (optional)

Process all ingredients until creamy, adding a little water if needed. Pour the mixture into wine or sundae glasses and chill in the fridge for thirty minutes. If you want this more like fudge, place in the freezer. This is a decadent pure chocolate treat that goes great at dinner parties

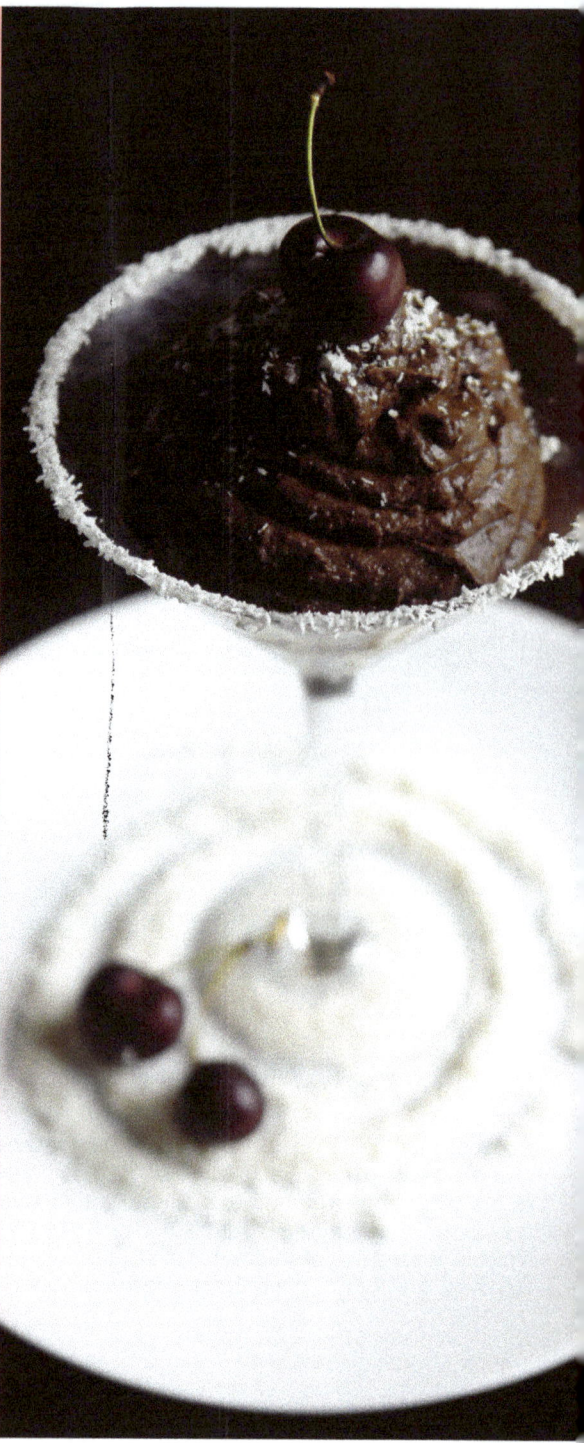

decadent cakes and pies ...

passionfruit cheesecake ...
makes 1 cake

base
1 cup of almond meal
½ cup of almonds
½ cup of pitted medjool dates
Mix all of the ingredients together and form into a dough. Press into a cake tin and put into the fridge to set

cake
½ cup of fresh lemon juice
3 tablespoons of yacon or agave syrup
1 tablespoon of coconut oil
1 tablespoon of pure vanilla extract
2 cups of pre-soaked cashews
2 tablespoons of lecithin granules
To make the cake, process lemon juice, cashews, natural sweetener, vanilla and coconut oil until creamy. Add in the lecithin at the end to thicken. Pour into the cake tin and let set in the freezer or fridge

topping
6 passionfruits or 3 mangoes
1 banana
1 tablespoon of natural sweetener

Remove the insides of the passionfruit and blend with banana and natural sweetener. Add a little water if needed. Pour over the top of the set cheesecake and place back in the freezer to set. If you want a mango cheesecake, simply use mangoes instead.

double choc beet cake ...
makes 1 large cake

cake
2 cups of almonds (soaked for 5 to 6 hours)
½ cup of cocoa powder
(or cacao if you want richer and healthier)
2 beetroots, grated
½ cup of pitted medjool dates
(or ¼ cup of agave, yacon or other)
½ cup of nut butter or tahini
1 teaspoon of pure vanilla
2 tablespoons of lecithin granules
1 tablespoon of lucuma or mesquite powder
a little purified water

icing (optional)
¼ cup of cocoa powder
¼ cup of cacao powder
2 avocadoes, mashed
1 tablespoon of lucuma powder
¼ cup of agave, yacon, stevia or pitted dates

This cake is really yummy on its own. If you feel like a completely decadent treat, then make the icing to go on top. To make the cake soak almonds and then blend in a food processor with cocoa or cacao, beetroot, natural sweetener, nut butter, lecithin, lucuma or mesquite, vanilla and water. Pour the mixture into a cake tin and freeze. To make the icing process ingredients until creamy and pour over the top of the cake. Place back in the fridge to set.

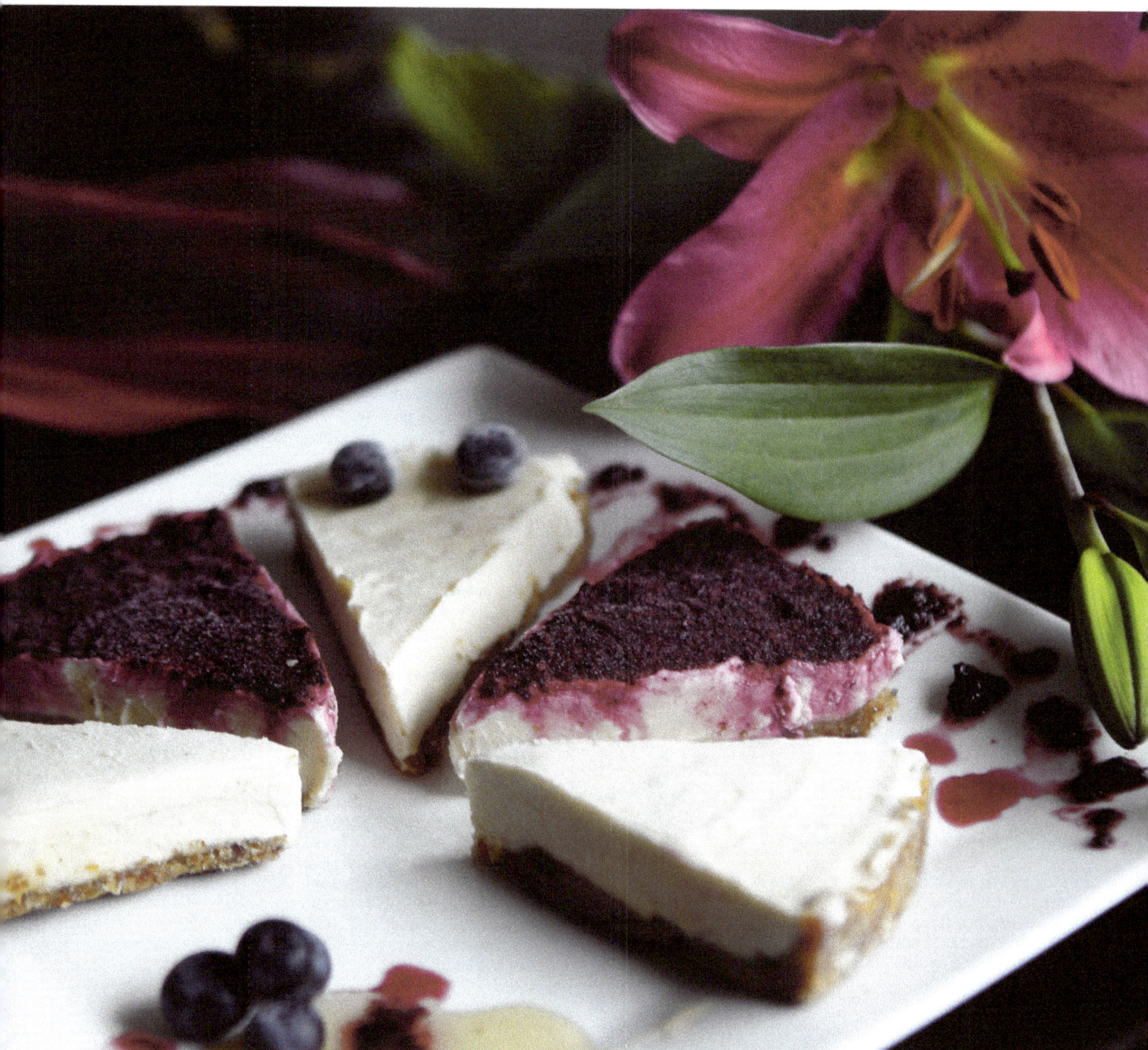

blueberry cheesecake ...

crust
2 cups of macadamia nuts
10 pitted medjool dates or ½ cup pitted dates
¼ cup of dessicated coconut or coconut meat
Process all of the ingredients together until it forms a dough like texture. Then press into a round tin.

cheesecake
2 cups of cashews, (pre-soaked)
4 lemons, squeezed
¾ cup of agave syrup or ½ cup of pitted dates (or other natural sweetener)
½ teaspoon of pure vanilla extract or 1 vanilla bean
a pinch of sea salt
water as needed
Grind the cashews firstly into a powder. Add the rest of the ingredients and blend until smooth. Pour this mixture into the crust and place in the freezer. You can either add the blueberries to the cheesecake mix or make a blueberry sauce for the top.

blueberry sauce
1 punnet of blueberries
1 ripe banana
1 tablespoon of stevia or xylitol or coconut palm sugar or other
Puree all of the ingredients until smooth. Pour over the cheesecake layer. Chill in the freezer until ready.

blueberries - a true superstar

Blueberries are true antioxidant superstars. They contain countless cancer-protective antioxidants, tannins, chlorogenic acid, lutein, carotene and kaempferol. These antioxidants guard fiercely against free radical damage that cause cancer, cardiovascular disease, ageing and infections. Blueberries have shown amazing potential in their fight against breast, colon, esophageal and other types of cancer. On top of this, blueberries contain B vitamins to boost energy, copper to improve blood health, zinc and manganese to boost immunity and potassium to improve heart health. No wonder I love blueberries so much.

medjool dates – healthy or not?

Even though one medjool date contains 66 calories, they contain huge amounts of vitamins and minerals to improve health. They are a good source of vitamin C, B1, B2, B3, B5, B6 and Vitamin A. The B vitamins found in this big date boosts energy, digestion and immune function and the rich Vitamin A levels wards off infections and cancer. At least 15 different minerals are found in dates, including potassium, iron, magnesium and zinc. It is a good source of fluorine to protect against tooth decay and selenium to guard against cancer. Only four dates can supply 540 mg of potassium to prevent strokes, heart disease, irregular heart rhythm and high blood pressure. One date supplies 2 grams of fibre to help prevent colon and breast cancer. Even though one medjool date contains 16 grams of natural sugars, when making raw treats you only need to use small amounts of these.

raw chocolate pecan pie

crust

2 ½ cups of raw organic pecans
14 large pitted medjool dates
A little cacao butter
2 tablespoons of agave or yacon syrup
Process ingredients until you get a dough like texture
If you don't have medjool dates, use normal dates
Press into a cake tin and place in the fridge for one hour

pie

2 cups of organic pecans
1 tablespoon of vanilla extract
½ cup of purified water
¼ cup of cacao powder
¼ cup of cocoa powder
1 tablespoon of lucuma powder (optional)
1 tablespoon of mesquite powder (optional)
3 avocadoes
½ cup of pitted dates or 2 teaspoons of stevia or 2 tbsp's of yacon or other...

Blend all pie ingredients together in a food processor until creamy, adding a little water if necessary
Pour the pie mixture over the crust. Place in the freezer quickly to set, then remove to the fridge
This will last for three to five days in the fridge

decadent chocolate slice ...
makes 6 to 8 slices

crust
1 cup of almond meal
½ cup of almonds
2 tablespoons of cacao powder
¼ cup of cacao butter or coconut oil
¼ cup of agave or yacon syrup or other (optional)

To make the crust combine all ingredients in a processor. It should have a dough-like consistency. Press the dough into a seven inch pan. Chill in the fridge for at least one hour.

slice
1 cup of cocoa powder
¼ cup of cacao powder
1 avocado, mashed
½ cup of agave or yacon or 1 tbsp of stevia or other
1 teaspoon of pure vanilla extract
1 tablespoon of lucuma powder

Process all of the ingredients in a blender until nice and creamy. Pour over the crust and put back in the fridge to chill for another hour.

super slices and chocolate indulgence ...

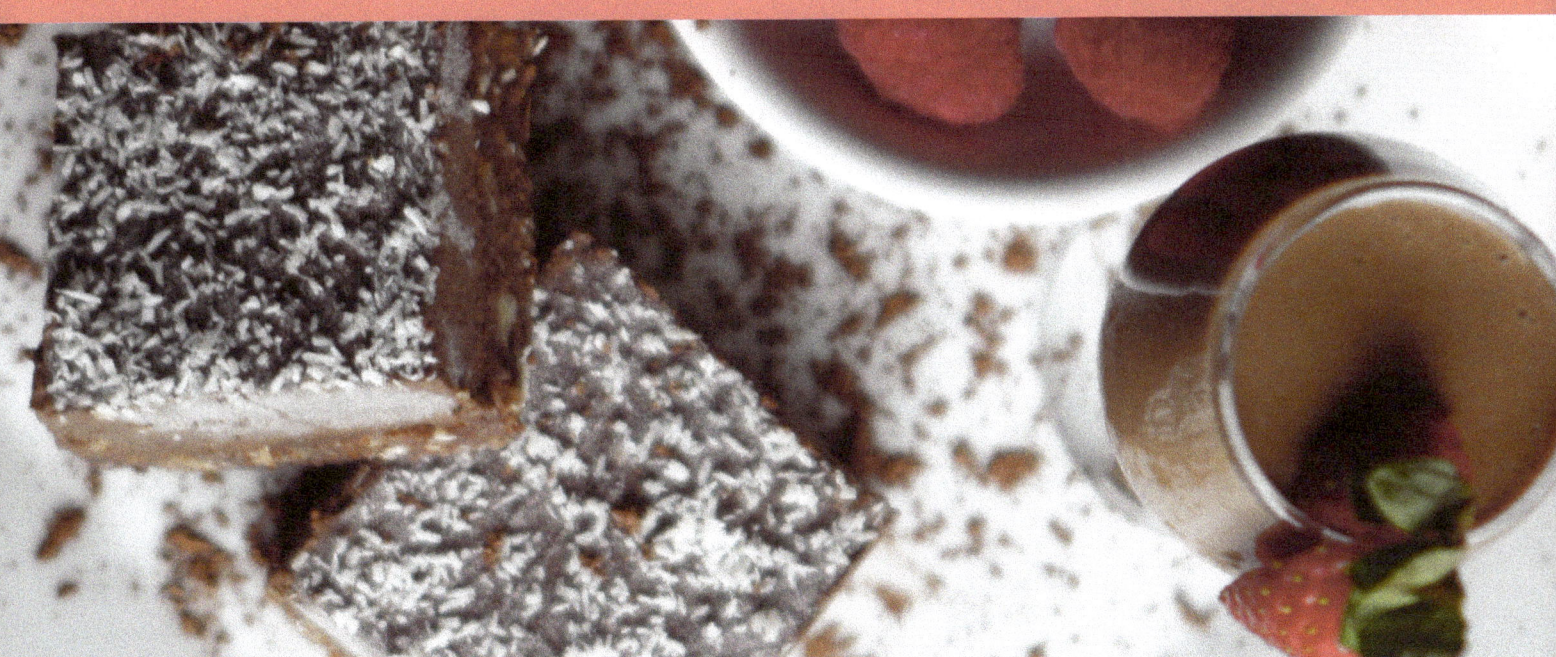

superfood chocolate truffles
makes 8 to 10 truffles

2 cups of cashews, grind down finely
½ to ¾ cup of pure cocoa or cacao powder
¼ cup of cacao butter
2 tablespoons of lucuma powder
1 tablespoon of mesquite powder
¼ cup of raw agave or yacon syrup or raw, unprocessed honey
¼ cup of desicated coconut or fresh coconut meat
¼ to ½ cup of purified water
(for blending – depending on desired texture)
1 teaspoon of pure vanilla extract
⅛ cup of your favourite superfood
(maca, colostrum, acai, green blend or other...)

Process ingredients until you get a nice and creamy texture. If you want your truffles more like milk chocolate, use cocoa powder. If you like the bitter taste of dark chocolate, use cacao powder or simply mix the two

chocolate to die for
makes around 16 chocolate pieces
1 inch thick each

1 cup of almonds
3 tablespoons of cocoa or cacao powder
4 tablespoons of coconut oil
1 chunk of cacao butter
2 tablespoons of lecithin granules
2 ¼ tablespoons of coconut palm sugar, xylitol or rapadura sugar (or alternative)
a little purified water

Process all of the ingredients until creamy, adding water to blend. Use a spatula and spread thinly in a tin and place in the freezer for 30 minutes. Remove, cut into one inch squares and place in the fridge in a container. You can change the flavour of this chocolate simply by adding different ingredients. I often swap the almonds for pistachio's and add fresh blueberries and coconut to make a pistachio and blueberry chocolate. To enhance the flavour add a little mesquite powder

CACAO
the heart smart love drug

Cacao powder is derived from the cacao bean. It contains powerful cancer-fighting and heart-protecting phytochemicals, as well as protein, fibre, iron, zinc, copper, calcium, magnesium and sulphur. The antioxidants found in cacao improve cardiovascular health by reducing clotting, improving circulation and blood pressure, lowering cholesterol and reducing the risk of strokes and heart attacks.

This magic powder can increase serotonin, a neurotransmitter that makes us feel positive, happy and peaceful. Cacao also stimulates endorphins to produce a 'pleasurable eurphoric' feeling and phenylethylamine – 'the LOVE chemical'. And if you thought that was enough, cacao also releases an amphetamine agent called anandamide. This substance provides us with feelings of happiness, bliss, excitement and that much sought after 'in love' feeling. No wonder we all like to indulge in chocolate when we are not feeling loved.

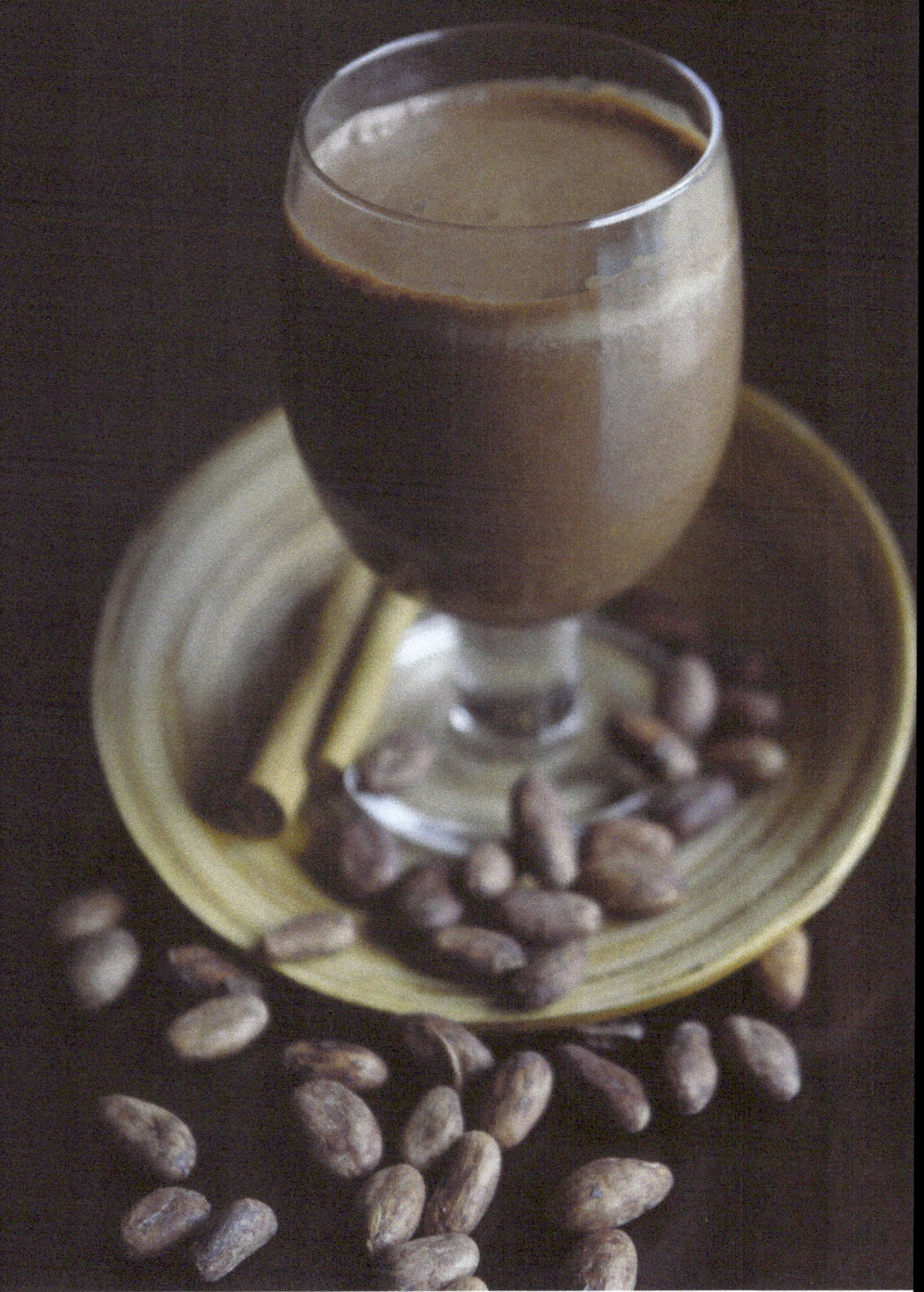

nutty choc balls
makes around 10 chocolate balls

Grind nuts in a food processor. Add the rest of the ingredients to the nut mix and roll into balls. Roll in shredded coconut. A very simple and nutritious treat!

1 cup of almond meal
1 cup of raw sunflower seeds
¼ cup of raw cashews
½ cup of raw hazelnuts
½ cup of tahini
½ cup of pitted medjool dates, agave, raw honey or maple syrup
¼ cup of cacao powder
¼ cup of cocoa powder
1 tablespoon of lucuma powder (optional)
1 tablespoon of mesquite powder (optional)
½ cup of dessicated or shredded coconut

fig fudge
makes 6 to 8 slices of fudge

Place cashews and hazelnuts in a blender with figs, natural sweetener, mesquite and avocado. Add a little water to mix well. Make into a paste and stir in flaxseed meal and water. Press into a tin and either freeze or put in the fridge. Cut into squares and store in the fridge or freezer. I love this fudge!

1 cup of cashews
1 cup of hazelnuts
½ cup of flaxseed meal
1 avocado
¼ cup of agave, yacon or maple syrup
(or 1 tbsp of xylitol, stevia or other)
¼ cup of cacao or cocoa powder
1 tablespoon of mesquite powder (optional)
½ cup of dried organic figs or fresh figs

vanilla goji balls
makes 10 to 12 balls

Process ingredients until you get a nice dough like texture Form into ball shapes and roll in sunflower seeds & refrigerate If you have time, soak nuts to soften

2 cups of macadamia nuts
¼ cup of flaxseed meal
½ cup of goji berries
½ cup of pitted medjool dates or yacon, agave or raw honey
¼ cup of tahini
2 tablespoons of lucuma or mesquite powder
1 vanilla bean or
1 teaspoon of pure vanilla extract
a handful of sunflower seeds

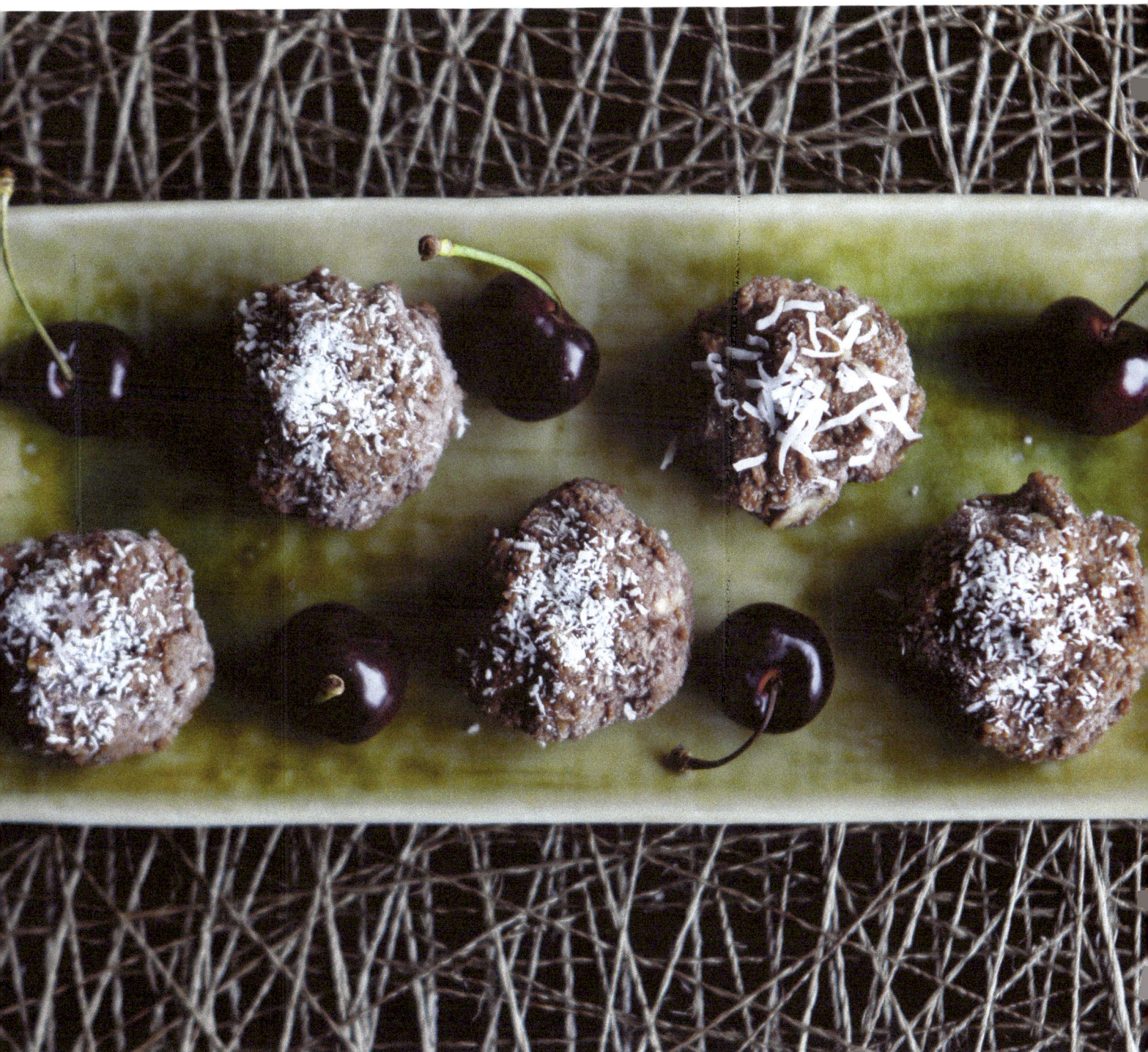

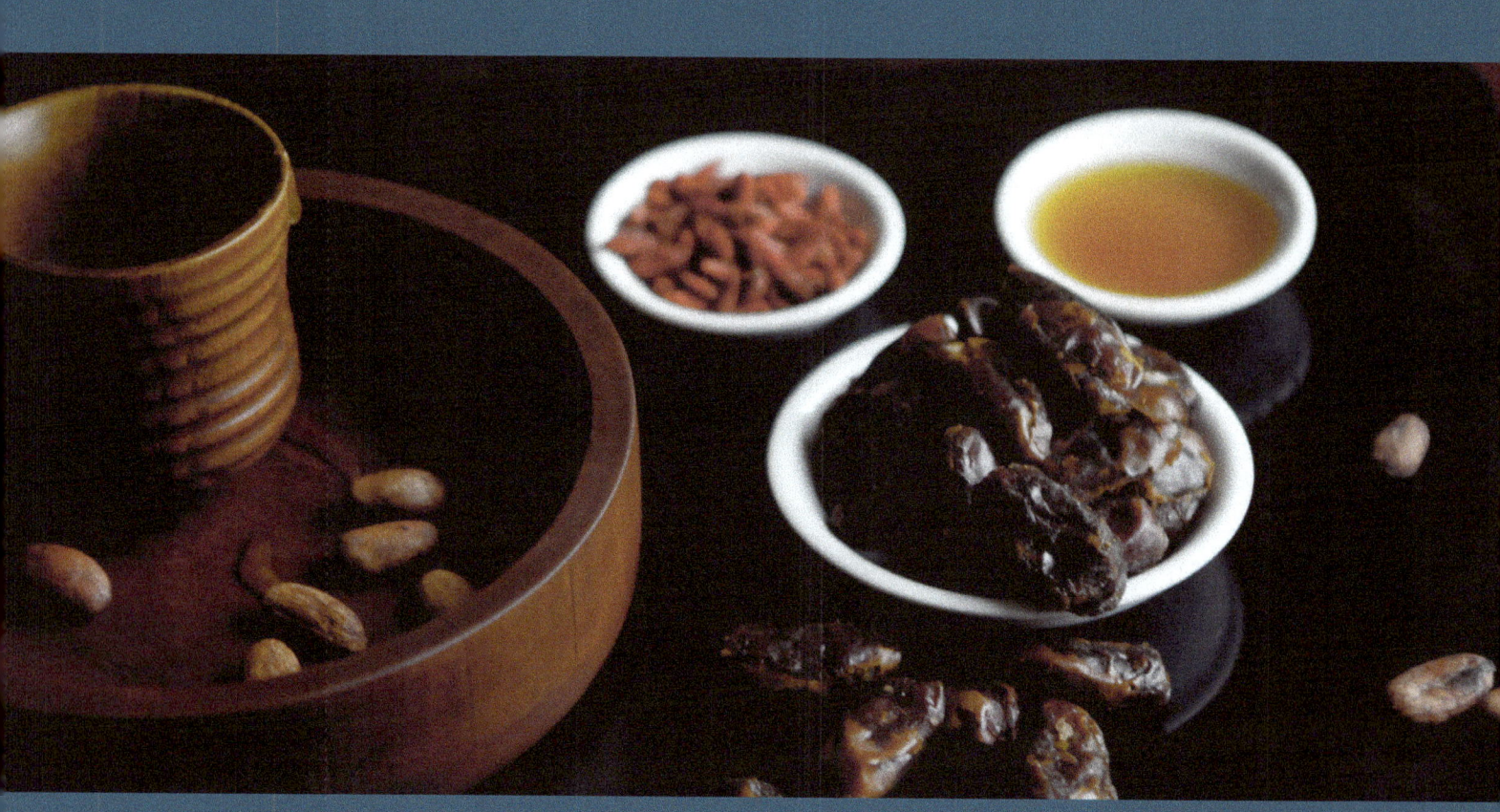

Shopping List ...

This shopping list will give you all of the ingredients to allow you to prepare every recipe within this book. There are certain ingredients like dried herbs and spices, oils and natural sweeteners that will last for a long time, so you will not need to buy regularly, whereas certain ingredients like fresh fruits and vegetables need to be bought fresh every week. This shopping list will tell you which ingredients I use most frequently to ensure they are always on hand to make the yummiest, raw living food dishes.

fresh vegetables ...

The most essential part of making raw foods in a 'living kitchen' is the incorporation of lots of fresh vegetables. I use raw vegetables in everything – even when I make dips, I cut up red capsicum, carrots, zucchini and celery and use these as my dipping tools. Vegetables should be the 'stars' in your raw food recipes. My favourite vegetables to use are:

Avocado
Baby spinach leaves
Beans – green
Bean sprouts
Beetroot
Bok choy
Broccoli
Cabbage (white and purple)
Capsicum – red and green
Carrots
Cauliflower
Celery
Corn cobs
Cucumber
Kale
Lettuce – romaine and mixed lettuce
Mushrooms – Baby bella, enoki, portabello
Olives – green and black (naturally dried – not lye cured)
Onions – white and Spanish
Peas – podded and snow
Radish
Rocket
Shitake mushrooms – fresh, (naturally log dried are also good)
Spring onions or shallots
Squash – winter
Tat soi
Tomatoes – roma, cherry and sun-dried
Watercress
Zucchini

fruits ...

Another equally essential ingredient found in 'living food recipes' is fresh fruit. Fruits are extremely cleansing and rejuvenating and supply huge amounts of minerals, antioxidants and vitamins. I repeatedly use these in special healing drinks, sweet treats, dips and even in salad dressings. If you are fighting cancer or you have a yeast problem, I wouldn't go overboard with fruit. Concentrate mainly on vegetable dishes and include some of the fruit recipes in moderation.

Apple (green and red)
Banana
Blueberries
Cherries
Coconuts (young and normal)
Goji berries (organic)
Grapes (purple are best)
Lemon
Limes
Mango
Paw Paw (green – for the green papaya salad and som tum salad)
Pears
Pineapple
Strawberries
Raspberries

fresh herbs and spices ...

I always have fresh herbs and spices on hand. I use them in most of my savoury dishes because of their amazing flavours, nutritional impact and healing qualities. Fresh herbs and spices are the 'key' to reversing complex diseases.

Basil
Coriander
Dill
Fennel
Galangal (used in a lot of the Asian dishes)
Garlic

Ginger root
Mint
Parsley
Red and Green Chilli (I love bird chilli's, jalapeno's and Thai chillies)
Rosemary
Thyme

dried herbs and spices ...

Luckily you do not have to buy these very often. They will last a long time in the cupboard and come in handy in case you run out of fresh herbs and you need to substitute with their dried counterpart.

Black Peppercorns (I also like green peppercorns)
Caraway seeds
Cayenne, ground
Chilli powder
Cinnamon, ground
Cumin, ground
Curry Powder or leaves
Lime leaves (Kaffir)
Mustard seeds
Nutmeg
Onion powder
Oregano
Paprika, ground
Rosemary
Thyme
Turmeric
Vanilla beans and/or liquid
Wasabi powder or paste

nuts and seeds ...

Nuts and seeds are the main ingredient in raw food dishes. They provide huge amounts of protein, minerals and essential fatty acids. I try to buy most of my nuts organic and store these in the fridge in glass jars. Most of these are pre-soaked to soften before using.

Almond
Brazil nut
Cashew
Chia seeds
Coconut, dried and shredded
Flaxseeds
Hazelnut
Macadamia
Pecans
Pine Nuts
Pistachio
Pumpkin seeds
Sesame seeds (white and black)
Sunflower seeds
Walnuts

natural butters ...

Cacao butter
Almond butter – you can make this yourself from almonds
Tahini (hulled or unhulled)

natural sweeteners...

All natural sweeteners should be raw and in their purest form. Choose the natural sweetener that suits your current health and lifestyle. Some sweeteners are much healthier than others with the healthiest options closest to the top.

Medjool dates
Stevia granules or powder
Erythritol granules or powder

Lucuma powder – expensive, but lasts a long time
Mesquite powder – expensive, but lasts a long time
Yacon syrup or Agave syrup (100% pure, raw, organic)
Xylitol (from birch trees) or organic corn
Raw unprocessed honey
Coconut palm sugar or rapadura sugar

salt and flavourings ...

Celtic Salt
Tamari (wheat free, low sodium)
Bragg's amino acid seasoning
Miso (I love shiro, but genmai and others are great too)
Fish Sauce (made from anchovies) – only if you are not vegan

natural oils ...

All the oils I buy are organic, undistilled, cold pressed and not exposed to heat or light.

Olive Oil (first cold pressed, extra virgin)
Sesame seed
Hemp seed
Flaxseed (needs to be cold pressed and refrigerated)
Coconut
Udo's oil
Macadamia, Walnut or others

vinegars ...

All the vinegars I buy are raw, undistilled and not exposed to heat or sunlight.

Apple Cider Vinegar - must contain the 'mother'
Balsamic vinegar
Brown rice vinegar
Red wine vinegar
Mirin

chocolate sweeteners ...

All the chocolate sweeteners I buy are in their purest form, organic, raw and not exposed to heat or light.

Cacao powder and nibs
Cocoa powder
Carob powder

grains ...

All grains should be organic, raw and in their purest forms.

Buckwheat groats
Lentils - green
Quinoa
Oat groats
Amaranth

seaweeds ...

Hijike (dried)
Arame (dried)
Kombu – (dried)
Dulse (red)

other ...

Almond meal
Coconut, dried and shredded
Flaxseed meal – should always be found in the fridge (otherwise it will be rancid)
Lecithin granules - at least 97% unbleached
Mustard paste – if you don't want to use the seeds
Nutritional yeast
Super foods – to boost up special drinks
Tofu – organic and GMO free – optional in dishes
Miso - genmai, shiro or others
Hulled hemp seeds

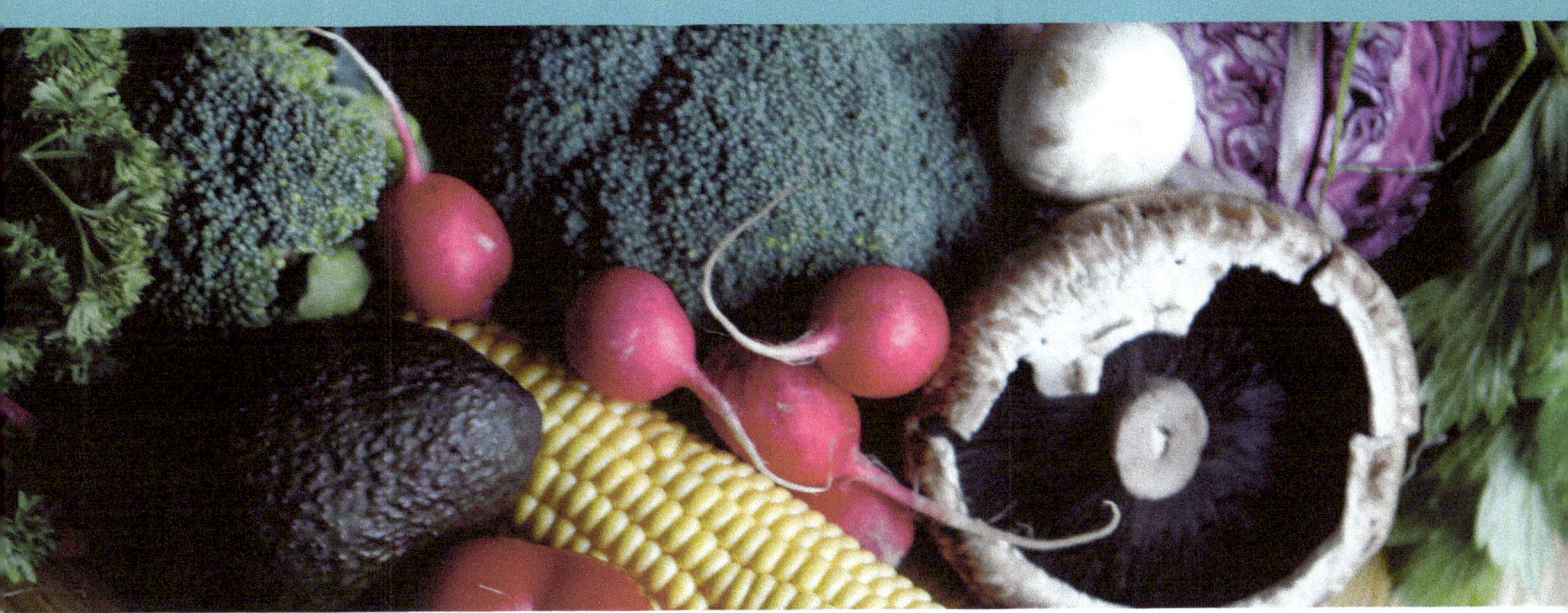

About Katrina and her centre...

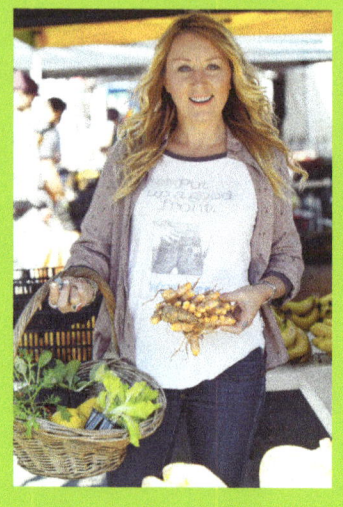

I grew up on the beautiful Tweed Coast of Australia with its spectacular beaches, healthy outdoor lifestyle and down-to-earth Australian people. As a little girl, I was quite a tomboy. My dad and brothers taught me how to ride motorbikes and skateboards, play football and how to surf, at the beautiful Byron Bay pass. That was in the days when Byron Bay only had a handful of streets, an ice-cream parlour where we challenged each other to pac-man and space invaders, a bowls club and plenty of open spaces to ride our bikes around on. Growing up in Australia was definitely an idyllic lifestyle and it taught me about the beauty of our natural surroundings and the absolute necessity to preserve these for my children.

Being a qualified naturopath, iridologist, herbalist and lecturer for close to twenty years I have had the honour to consult with many inspirational people including famous movie stars, politicians, musicians, company directors and royalty from all over the globe. My love of writing has allowed me to publish many health and motivational books, including an international best seller - 'Shattering the Cancer Myth'. To date, 'Raw Addiction' has been one of my most exciting books to create. It allowed me to experiment with the tantalizing flavours of local Australian produce and in doing so create an assortment of simple, delicious and wholesome raw food creations – all designed to transform health. This book drew me back to the beauty of my country and made me realise how important it is to fight for our farmers, our land, our animals and our right to eat clean foods.

When I'm not cooking up a 'raw food storm' I spend my time with kids surfing, writing and consulting in my natural health centre at 'Kirra'. This centre is a 'hub of positivity, inspiration and wellness' run by a team of healthy, beautiful souls. Here we offer 'real life tools' to help each person find their true health and happiness. My website www.katrinaellis.com.au gives free information, advice and directions on how to find the 'best of everything' in regards to health and healing. I am constantly writing new books, presenting motivational seminars and updating my centre's technology to offer the best tools possible to change lives for the better. For more information, visit the website or call our centre on +61 7 5536 3113.

Wishing you good health, happiness and peace,
Katrina x

Thanks....

This is my favourite part of the book where I get to thank the people I love for their support and patience. To Clay-Jay and my beautiful, awesome kids, Carter and Evie-Ray thanks for being my taste testing guinea pigs...

To my beautiful mum Ann and my amazing dad Hedley (thanks for giving me such a fun, free, adventurous and loving upbringing) – these gifts have given me the courage to share my ideas with the world. I also want to thank my caring brothers Larry and Brett (dad would be proud, just like I am), my lifelong friends Roderick, Justin and Roland, my mentor and friend Dr Michael Hayter, the beautiful Mr Andy, the incredible, super-organised Miss Danni, all my wonderful clients and friends who teach me something new every day and Carter's best friend Beau – who wondered why I didn't mention him in my other books!

Lastly, but definitely not least, I want to thank Mish for dedicating hours of her time to making the design of this book unique and fresh! Hey Mish – just a personal note – "Don't you ever leave me.........cause I'll find you!!!" (ha ha...)

www.ingramcontent.com/pod-product-compliance
Ingram Content Group UK Ltd.
Pitfield, Milton Keynes, MK11 3LW, UK
UKHW051351180426
11947UKWH00014B/869